AI-Powered IoT for
COVID-19

AI-Powered IoT for COVID-19

Fadi Al-Turjman

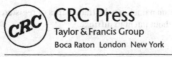

CRC Press
Taylor & Francis Group
Boca Raton London New York

CRC Press is an imprint of the
Taylor & Francis Group, an **informa** business

First Edition published [2021]
by CRC Press
6000 Broken Sound Parkway NW, Suite 300, Boca Raton, FL 33487-2742

and by CRC Press
2 Park Square, Milton Park, Abingdon, Oxon, OX14 4RN

© 2021 Taylor & Francis Group, LLC

CRC Press is an imprint of Taylor & Francis Group, LLC

ISBN: 978-0-367-56674-6 (hbk)
ISBN: 978-1-003-09888-1 (ebk)

Typeset in Times
by Deanta Global Publishing Services, Chennai, India

Dedication

You might need a doctor to diagnose a disease, however, you need somebody who care to recognize suffering. And for sure, the struggle you are facing today is developing the strength you need for tomorrow.

This book is dedicated for those who are suffering and in need for support.. and for those who care and are welling to support.

To the beauty in my life... to my wonderful family.

Fadi Al-Turjman

Contents

Preface

Coronavirus, or COVID-19, has significantly affected daily life around the globe. It emphasized the real need for interconnected devices and enabling technologies via what we call the Internet of Things (IoT) paradigm. This tightly integrates with the existing Cloud infrastructure to impact several COVID-19–affected fields. Intelligent IoT-enabled COVID-19 solutions have made revolutionary advances in all these fields, and in the biomedical field specifically. It finds more appropriate and accurate diagnosis that eliminates the demerits of traditional methods, which can involve significant human errors and/or inaccuracy. Moreover, it reduces the time for the disease diagnosis, detection, and treatment. This book opens the door for several exciting research topics and applications in this era. In this book, we are resolving significant issues towards realizing the future vision of Artificial Intelligence (AI) in IoT-enabled spaces. AI-powered IoT solutions have been employed in fighting one of the most critical pandemics, COVID-19, towards further advances in our daily smart life. This book overviews the associated issues and proposes the most up-to-date alternatives. The objective is to pave the way for AI-powered IoT-enabled spaces in next generation technologies and open the door for further innovative ideas.

Fadi Al-Turjman

About the Author

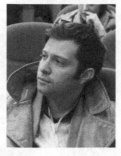 **Prof. Dr. Fadi Al-Turjman** received his PhD in computer science from Queen's University, Kingston, Ontario, Canada, in 2011. He is a full professor and a research center director at Near East University, Nicosia, Cyprus. Prof. Al-Turjman is a leading authority in the areas of smart/intelligent, wireless, and mobile networks' architectures, protocols, deployments, and performance evaluation. His publication history spans over 250 publications in journals, conferences, patents, books, and book chapters, in addition to numerous keynotes and plenary talks at flagship venues. He has authored and edited more than 25 books about cognition, security, and wireless sensor networks' deployments in smart environments, published by Taylor & Francis Group, Elsevier, and Springer. He has received several recognitions and best papers' awards at top international conferences. He also received the prestigious *Best Research Paper Award* from Elsevier Computer Communications Journal for the period 2015–2018, in addition to the *Top Researcher Award* for 2018 at Antalya Bilim University, Turkey. Prof. Al-Turjman has led a number of international symposia and workshops in flagship communication society conferences. Currently, he serves as an associate editor and the lead guest/associate editor for several well-reputed journals, including the *IEEE Communications Surveys and Tutorials* (**IF 22.9**) and the Elsevier *Sustainable Cities and Society* (**IF 4.7**).

List of Contributors

Motaz Alawna
Department of Physiotherapy and
  Rehabilitation
School of Health Sciences
Istanbul Gelisim University
Istanbul, Turkey

and

Department of Physiotherapy and
  Rehabilitation
Arab American University
Jenin, Palestine

Vishal Bhardwaj
Bharati Vidyapeeth's College of
  Engineering
New Delhi, India

Gopal Chaudhary
Bharati Vidyapeeth's College of
  Engineering
New Delhi, India

Ekansh Chauhan
Maharaja Agrasen Institute of
  Technology
New Delhi, India

Pwadubashiyi Pwavodi Coston
Research Centre for AI and IoT
Near East University
Nicosia, Turkey

Barakat A. Dawood
Computer Engineering Dept.
and
Research Centre for AI and IoT
Near East University
Nicosia, Turkey

Basil Bartholomew Duwa
Department of Biomedical Engineering
Research Center for AI and IoT
Near East University
Nicosia, Turkey

N. Gayathri
School of Computing Science and
  Engineering
Galgotias University
Greater Noida, Uttar Pradesh, India

Deepak Gupta
Maharaja Agrasen Institute of
  Technology
New Delhi, India

Adedoyin A. Hussain
Computer Engineering Dept.
and
Research Centre for AI and IoT
Near East University
Nicosia, Turkey

Abdullahi Umar Ibrahim
Research Centre for AI and IoT
Near East University
Nicosia, Turkey

Rahul Jain
Bharati Vidyapeeth's College of
  Engineering
New Delhi, India

Ashish Khanna
Maharaja Agrasen Institute of
  Technology
New Delhi, India

Puneet Singh Lamba
Bharati Vidyapeeth's College of
    Engineering
New Delhi, India

Ayman A Mohamed
Department of Physiotherapy and
    Rehabilitation
School of Health Sciences
Istanbul Gelisim University
Istanbul, Turkey

and

Department of Basic Sciences
Faculty of Physical Therapy
Beni-Suef University
Beni Suef, Egypt

Majdi Nassif
Department of Physiotherapy and
    Rehabilitation
Arab American University
Jenin, Palestine

Muhammad Hassan Nawaz
Electrical Engineering Dept.
University of Debrecen
Debrecen, Hungary

Mehmet Ozsoz
Department of Biomedical
    Engineering
Research Center for AI and IoT
Near East University
Nicosia, Turkey

S. Punitha
Department of Computer Science and
    Engineering
Karunya Institute of Technology and
    Sciences
Coimbatore, India

S. Rakeshkumar
School of Computing Science and
    Engineering
Galgotias University
Greater Noida, Uttar Pradesh, India

Prerit Rathi
Bharati Vidyapeeth's College of
    Engineering
New Delhi, India

Rajat Sharma
Bharati Vidyapeeth's College of
    Engineering
New Delhi, India

Prateek Singal
Bharati Vidyapeeth's College of
    Engineering
New Delhi, India

Manpreet Sirswal
Maharaja Agrasen Institute of
    Technology
New Delhi, India

Deepanshu Srivastava
School of Computing Science and
    Engineering
Galgotias University
Greater Noida, Uttar Pradesh, India

Thompson Stephan
Department of Computer Science and
    Engineering, Faculty of Engineering
    and Technology, M. S. Ramaiah
    University of Applied Sciences
Bangalore, India

Vishal Tyagi
Bharati Vidyapeeth's College of
    Engineering
New Delhi, India

1 Cloud Computing and Business Intelligence in IoT-Enabled Smart and Healthy Cities

Barakat A. Dawood, Fadi Al-Turjman,
and Muhammad Hassan Nawaz

CONTENTS

1.1   INTRODUCTION

In recent times, there have been major talks about cloud computing (CC). Currently, large numbers of organizations are processing an enormous number of exchanges to break down, oversee, and produce powerful data for business choices which turn out to be better, yet these exchanges take various volumes of information and are hard to oversee. Associations need to monitor their business information every year, as the measure of value-based information is quickly increasing by digitally generating, capturing, and storage processing. Various sectors subsequently use this idea of technology efficiently [1, 2]; integration is on-demand in areas like Business Intelligence (BI), which is still associated with numerous difficulties [3]. Majorly, individuals see this technology to have more possibility in transforming a huge portion of the industry concerning IT [4]. Cloud computing can be a board framework system and a business conveyance model. In the aspect of business delivery, this model provides the user or individual with experiences in ways such as hardware and software, and also resources related to the network are excellent leverage in giving innovation to administrations over the internet, and servers will be given in respect of the lucid needs by the organization using improved, computerized instruments [5]. The internet boosts the development of cloud computing technology continuously. In the previous decade, there were certain stages where software solutions took over traditional hardware architecture; this was attainable due to the evolution of Business Intelligence systems. Saying traditional, this relates to a simplified model which organizations used for information in-house on a server or numerous cuts off, and dealt with it with the current programming. A complex outline of business processes is offered by Business Intelligence solutions these days. Software that can give procedures, stockpiling, and investigations of information from different offices is being integrated. The holistic way of building and running an integrated management support system or infrastructure is being characterized by Business Intelligence. The need for a greater amount of heterogeneous systems is being raised due to the wide range of tasks [6]. Over a while, it is said that the systems evolve into a complex and highly integrated BI architecture [7]. However, cloud computing, which is a new technology, permanently poses new infrastructural challenges [8]. Integrating specialized software is not just the ability of a business solution, it also comprises building a custom equipment engineering that will have the option to deal with processes arising from activities by the software. The traditional way of life of humans is changing due to the combined methodology of large information and distributed computing, which brings new open doors for the development of organizations in online business. Web-based business endeavors open ways to new developments in business and advances with distributed computing abilities in the vital rising ventures, and legislature accordingly gave a few strategies to help this development. Enormous organizations are making stage-based, web-based business frameworks by utilizing databases, huge information, and distributed computing advancements. This has numerous points of interest on business knowledge and impact on distributed computing advances. Distributed computing welcomes numerous points of interest in business and manufactures more astute lives for individuals. Utilizing cloud computing, cost-effective solutions are experienced by organizations. This will minimize the pressure on their financial planning with regards to investments in comparison to the old-style model, where organizations depended on server farms and the support identified with such. Pretty much every zone, with the usage of programming arrangements and with the utilization of cloud computing condition, is an addition to organizations.

1.1.1 COMPARISON TO OTHER SURVEYS

There are abundant differing perceptions of the expression of distributed computing rotating around a perspective view. While in the cloud it is commonly just seen as boundless computer resources accessible on-demand [9], there likewise exists an increasingly refined method that builds up distributed computing as another model in IT sourcing that helps smoothness and encourages new plans of action. An all-around utilized clarification deciphers distributed processing as a model for completing unavoidable, invaluable, on-request sort out approach to bargain with a typical pool of constructible figuring assets that can be quickly provisioned and circulated [10, 11]. The administrations given through the cloud regularly change in the middle of the inventory of fundamental processing assets (IaaS) up to the provision of the sophisticated platform (PaaS) or application software (SaaS) [12, 13].

BI service administration (BISA) is a modification of IT service organization (ITSA), which is created from the growing entanglement of IT frameworks to uphold an increasingly intelligible idea to improve flexibility and precision of the IT environment [14]. In this manner, it tends to be typified as depicting, overseeing, and discharging IT administrations to support business goals and client necessities [6], whereas the specified service world symbolizes a mixture of technology, people, and procedures. This description analyzes the more comprehensive organizational role of service administration and therefore, distinctly differentiates it from exclusively technical service-oriented architecture (SOA) method [3]. Besides, service administration infrastructure utilized in performing, such as ITIL or COBIT, now and again includes valuable ideas to configure, watch, and oversee administrations [15].

1.1.2 Scope of the Paper and Its Contribution

Cloud computing is a model for business conveyance and a system support strategy. The model for business conveyance gives clients involvement with which equipment, programming, and system assets are astoundingly impacted to deliver inventive administrations over the Web, and servers are prepared by the coherent necessities of the administration utilizing dynamic, automated hardware. The cloud permits administration makers, program executives, and others to utilize these administrations through a Web-based system that extricates the entanglements of the key unique structure. The structure upkeep strategy permits IT foundations to keep up enormous quantities of extraordinary virtual assets as a solitary incredible asset [16]. It additionally permits IT associations to extend their server farm assets hugely, with no critical increment in the number of individuals expected to deal with the development. For foundations, and by utilizing the regular structure, the cloud will permit clients to assimilate IT assets in the server farm in a new example that was never accessible. Organizations that work the customary server farm upkeep rehearsals realize that accessibility of IT assets to an end client can be time thorough. It requires numerous procedures, for example, equipment obtainment; finding raised floor space and force and cooling adequacy; assignment of heads to introduce working frameworks, middleware and programming; organizing provisioning; and security of the encompassing. Most organizations have found that this procedure can take up to a few months. The IT foundations that re-arrange existing equipment assets find that, despite everything, it takes a little while to accomplish. Cloud viably facilitates this test by actualizing computerization, business work processes, and asset separation that empowers a client to surf through an index of IT administrations, add the administrations to their shopping basket, and recognize the request.

After the request has been endorsed by an executive, the cloud finishes the procedure. This methodology lessens the necessary time to make the assets accessible to the client inside a shorter term. Right now, we present an outline for BI and spotlight on the procedures to be considered while managing the difficulties presented by BI in the cloud.

In this work, we can outline our commitments as follows:

- We overview BI in the cloud in detail.
- We outline the key structural factors that are required when running BI in the cloud.
- We categorize the different procedures in BI.
- We outline the used information technology concerning the cloud and BI.
- We abridge the primary open research issues and difficulties in this paper.

The organization of the paper is as per the following. In Section 1.2, we overview the fundamental contribution in cloud computing-related territory, the primary parts, and system design, and it gives a short prologue to cloud computing. Section 1.3 shows the design elements of cloud computing (CC) and business intelligence (BI). Scholarly overviews exhibited in writing and illustrating methods in BI and cloud computing are examined in Section 1.4. Section 1.5 reviews the key empowering advances utilized in data innovation in the cloud and BI. Section 1.6 talks about the intelligent areas in the cloud and BI. Section 1.7 describes cloud IoT in combatting COVID-19. Section 1.8 talks about the security, while Section 1.9 talks about the potential hazards of cloud BI adoption. Section 1.10 emphasizes discussion, outlines open research issues in BI and the cloud, and features future research patterns. At last, Section 1.11 closes our survey, which has been presented in this survey. For greater intelligibility, Table 1.1 gives an outline of the abbreviations used and their definitions.

1.2 CLOUD COMPUTING

Distributed computing can be characterized as the game plan of processing administrations (servers, stockpiling, databases, systems, programming, investigation, knowledge, and so on) over the web through the cloud to keep up faster modernization, customizable assets, and size of the economy [17]. Users regularly only need to pay for the cloud services as they are used; this helps in reduction of functional costs, efficient running of the infrastructure, and scope, as the business requires changing [18]. Distributed computing produces figuring, stockpiling, administrations, and applications over the web [19]. For a smart phone to be energy effective and computationally efficient, main adjustments in hardware and software levels are often necessary. Distributed computing can essentially be characterized as representing a merge of frameworks that are linked together into a network, and contributes an extensible framework for software systems and data to make use of. Through the use of this result, the cost of software results,, implementation and data storage is drastically reduced. To understand better what is represented by distributed computing, we have to relate it to customary speculations, for instance, grid computing, as depicted in Figure 1.1.

TABLE 1.1

Abbreviations Used

Terms	Meaning
AI	Artificial Intelligence
API	Application Program Interfaces
APT	Advanced Persistent Threat
BI	Business Intelligence
CFL	Compact Fluorescent Lamps
CRM	Customer Relationship Management
DoS	Denial of Service
DSS	Decision Support Systems
DTD	Document Type Data
ERP	Enterprise Resource Planning
IaaS	Infrastructure as a Service
IP	Internet Protocol
IT	Information Technology
ML	Machine Learning
OLAP	Online Analytical Processing
PaaS	Platform as a Service
SaaS	Software as a Service
TCP	Transmission Control Protocol

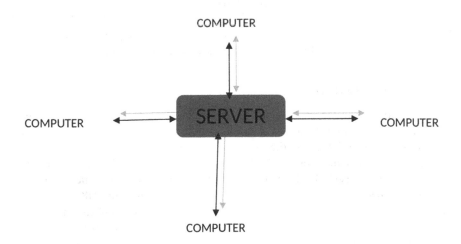

FIGURE 1.1   Grid computing.

Grid Computing in Figure 1.1 depicts the use of assets from numerous PCs connected in a system to carry out just a single issue at once. The test with network processing is that if there is disappointment in one framework, there is a high danger of disillusionment for the others. Distributed computing in Figure 1.2 endeavors to overcome this test by utilizing all the frameworks in the system to such an extent that

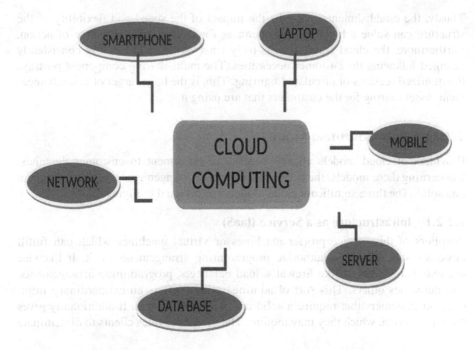

FIGURE 1.2 Technology of cloud computing.

if there is disappointment in one framework, it will naturally be supplanted. Grid computing has the goal that the assets can be utilized to tackle a solitary issue. The systems that are a piece of such structures can be dispersed everywhere throughout the globe. In any case, in a relationship with grid computing, distributed computing can be characterized as a created network registering structure.

Cloud assets can be re-appropriated on request to address the issues of the customer. For example, in certain nations, clients are not permitted to store information past their limit. To have the option to accomplish that, suppliers of cloud administrations can make a system that can live in that nation. Additionally, the cloud system can be flexible and can accommodate cases and different time zones to implement with. If the cloud result is organized in Canada, it might be used by European clients, since it can adjust to grouped time zones [20].

1.2.1 Cloud Computing Characteristics

Concerning the consequences of the cloud, it can be characterized as having tremendous adaptability, ability, colossal chance and reliability, and multi-sharing. As respects, the colossal versatility includes, enabling the usage of advantages for innumerable customers that have different requests [21]. The ability highlighted portrays the critical time of the framework with respect to the assignments proposed by clients. Considering this case, the analysis time is extraordinarily short, seeing how complex the structure is. A cloud structure is significantly available and dependable.

Thusly, the establishments that take the impact of the speed and flexibility of the structure can value a high pace of openness for their cultivated course of action. Furthermore, the cloud framework is truly trustworthy, because it is consistently changed following the customer necessities. The multi-sharing component portrays the itemized sections of circulated figuring. This is the huge target of this advancement: asset sharing for the customers that are using it.

1.2.2 CLOUD COMPUTING MODELS

Providers of cloud models convey benefits in agreement to customer demands. Concerning these models, the accomplished cloud arrangements are price proficient and solid. The three significant cloud models are depicted in Figure 1.3.

1.2.2.1 Infrastructure as a Service (IaaS)

Suppliers of this service proffer machines or virtual machines which can fulfill customer solicitations to authorize programming arrangements on it. It likewise presents various assets like firewalls, load balancers, programming arrangements, and numerous others. This sort of administration proffers an extraordinary influence on customers that require a solid and adaptable system. It additionally gives them protection, which they may require. The model provides clients to disseminate

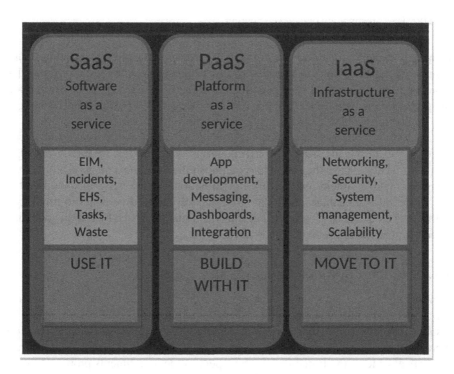

FIGURE 1.3 Models of computing in the cloud.

their products with sponsored rates. An extra advantage of utilizing IaaS is that customers can disseminate and continue the working arrangement of the system. Thusly, the supplier isn't pressuring the customers to utilize any particular OS [22]. Fundamentally, these customers pay only for the assets they utilized for their accomplished arrangement, without fretting over equipment support.

1.2.2.2 Platform as a Service (PaaS)

The service has just introduced a working framework, a programmable language, and a web server, etc. Likely, it is a generally utilized kind of model, since it advances the presentation and confirmation of programming results. This model likewise presents the necessary assets for an application to work viably. The assets are immediately allotted with the goal that the client doesn't need to physically do that [23].

1.2.2.3 Software as a Service (SaaS)

In the model, it is clarified to be a compensation as-you-use model that the vendors offer to customers a customized (machines and programming) arrangement. To get to this, customers should pay for membership. The upside of utilizing the framework is that customers never have to make a big deal about any equipment or programming support. The SaaS provider manages that for the customer [23]. For a nitty-gritty perspective, SaaS can offer entry for an establishment to a BI course of action. For this, the establishment will pay a month to month or yearly enrollment due that will be constrained by the customization of the BI plan and also the benefits appropriated to that establishment.

1.2.3 CLOUD DEPLOYMENT MODEL

There are three significant kinds of cloud organization models. In Table 1.2, we portray their criteria.

1.2.3.1 Public Cloud

The public cloud conventionally infers that it is visible for the open use. Customers can save data on it with no insurance, like a protected framework. This kind of cloud is likewise offered as free for general use. The significant stress is security, since suppliers can't give affirmation of it [24].

TABLE 1.2

Cloud Deployment Models

Area	Private Cloud	Hybrid Cloud	Public Cloud
Cost	Depends on the assigned resources	Lesser than Private Cloud	Free
Security	Very secure	Moderately secure	Low
Flexibility	High	High	High
Resources	Depends on user requirements	Depends on user requirements	High

1.2.3.2   Private Cloud

The system is utilized uniquely inside one establishment. It can be constructed whether it is in an establishment premise (server center) or gotten to through the supplier. This is an extremely secure cloud model that is favored by most establishments since, when it is constructed remotely, the supplier offers support administration [24]. An extra advantage is that the assets are allotted to a solitary customer. With this, the structure is usually worked to convey incredible viability and security.

1.2.3.3   Hybrid Cloud

The framework is the mix of the private and also the public cloud models. However, customers can show what data stays an open cloud and what stays private. The benefit of using a hybrid cloud is thus the sponsored cost [25].

1.2.3.4   Community Cloud

There is, additionally, the fourth sort of cloud sending model, which is known as the Community Cloud. This alludes to a cloud system utilized by a gathering of foundations inside a similar area that conveys information on it. This sort of structure is utilized by government parastatals, colleges from a region or even a nation, providers, and so on [25]. The security offered by this sort of deployment is essentially the same as the deployment of a private cloud, since it is a private cloud that is divided by different substances with basic goals.

1.2.4   RESTRICTIONS AND OPPORTUNITIES OF CLOUD COMPUTING

The limitations of CC can be ordered in the type of reception, development, business, and strategy [26]. The primary limitation expected to vanquish in cloud computing is information security. A great many people believe that keeping information on a common structure realizes a protection issue. They even feel that information must be seen with certain products under certain security conditions, for example, secret key ensured, encryption, and so on, yet this isn't adequate. The cloud client takes the weight for the security of the product that he empowered in the cloud environment. This is a test because, in a shut and controlled structure, for example, intranet, the client can just move toward the framework from inside the system. Arrangements like this can keep up enough security since it can't be drawn nearer remotely from the confided in organization. The cloud can't do that, in as much as the specialist co-op guarantees the security of the system by extra firewalls and other equipment or programming arrangements that blocks pariahs from information burglary. This is successful much of the time, however, there are circumstances in which cloud customers are setback by phishing goals and messages. For instance, if an association uses a changed BI engaged in the cloud to which its workers login just with the username and mystery express, then anyone that approaches those capabilities can log in into the structure. Tragically, customers are not continually aware, and potentially they use uncomplicated or piddling passwords, or they complete phishing structures. At present, the provider can't accept obligation. If the security of the cloud structure is hurt, data from various clients may be revealed to chance. Another security issue is to shield the customer from the provider. This proposes the provider can see all the data that is gotten a good deal on the structure and do anything he needs with it, even though it is illicit. To keep customers secure from that, they can utilize programming that empowers them to encode significant information [27]. By so doing, regardless of whether the supplier can see the information, he can't utilize it, since he can't understand it. By information encryption, the client may experience a few troubles in the critical time of the empowered programming, because the data is encoded on one side and moved to the cloud system like in Figure 1.4. This strategy must be switched so the client can peruse the data. Another limitation in the utilization of distributed computing is getting programming authorization. Programming providers conventionally sell their items with a grant. Since in the cloud there is a surge of machines that are working at the same time, this kind of grant isn't fitting. Cloud providers, with everything taken into account, use open source programming. Programming engineers are beginning to change over their grant understanding with the objective that the item they organized can be useable in a cloud area.

1.2.5 CLOUD COMPUTING QUALITIES

Comparable to all technologies, the technology of the cloud has some qualities that regulate its capacities. The qualities [27] are evaluated and compiled as listed below.

1.2.5.1 Storage over the Internet
This technique can be described as a technology structure that makes use of the Transmission Control Protocol/Internet Protocol (TCP/IP) network to get a connection

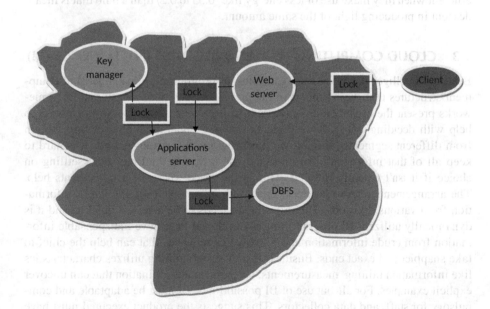

FIGURE 1.4 Data encryption to cloud computing.

with the servers and storage devices and to promote the storage solution arrangement. Storage on the internet is also referred to as Internet Protocol storage (IP storage) technology. By combining the best storage and networking industry methods, IP storage produces a huge performance and ascendable storage IP result [28].

1.2.5.2   Service over Internet

The fundamental aim of internet services is to assist customers all over the world to change their objectives into accomplishments by influencing the ability, speed, and pervasiveness of the internet [29].

1.2.5.3   Application Used over Internet

Using an internet connection, work on the server can also be done easily, instead of the program being installed on your computer, like the traditional program model. Cloud application is the application that is running on your local computer system when making use of cloud computing, or can scientifically be called an application running on the internet. Google Apps, Facebook, and Online Banking are examples [30] of powerful high-level programs that operate with incredible function ability for users who need a browser and internet connection.

1.2.5.4   Energy Efficiencies

Energy consumption management and inhibited growth is simply referred to as energy efficiency. This involves increasing energy efficiency by more service productivity for the same input of energy, or decreasing in energy for the same service for input [30]. For example, we take CFLs (compact fluorescent lamps) to be more efficient when they make use of less energy like (0.33 to 0.2) than a bulb that is incandescent in producing light of the same amount.

1.3   CLOUD COMPUTING (CC) AND BUSINESS INTELLIGENCE (BI)

Business Intelligence outlines the gathering of programming machines and equipment structures that show support in the precise arranging of a business. BI frameworks present the organization answers to collect, store, and assess information to help with deciding. Most establishments amass a gigantic amount of information from different segments utilizing various programming arrangements. It is hard to keep all of that information together and use it during the time spent settling on choice if it isn't recently filtrated. This is the place where BI arrangements help. The arrangements tend to proffer a rapid and fathomable examination of information from various divisions. The information tends to be assessed quickly, and it is dynamically utilized. BI programming is developed to remove indispensable information from crude information and to reveal experiences that can help the chief to take snappier and exact ends. Business insight programming utilizes characteristics like information mining, measurements, and prescient examination that can uncover explicit examples. For all-out use of BI possibilities, BI must be adaptable and compulsory for staff, and data collectors. This suggests the product executed must have the option to offer access to organized information for all the staff in connection with their profession. BI solutions are beneficial to prevail in competition [31]. With important information, it will help an establishment to approach its deficiencies and stabilities. Also, it is beneficial to make the right prognosis so that the authorities will reach resolutions that will assist the business to achieve its purpose, like in Figure 1.5.

Business Intelligence programming is fit to deliver all around archived reports to the specialists relying upon the data accumulated from various sources, either inside or remotely. Building an effective BI arrangement is additionally according to the significance of the prepared data. Working with crude information devours a great deal of time, and it is moderately troublesome. To forestall investigations of immaterial information, the perfect arrangement is to utilize specially constructed programming for every division that is influenced during the time spent on the business. After this reason for existing is achieved, the BI arrangement empowered will create real outcomes. In the organizational procedure of Business Intelligence software, there are excessive dangers including: framework plan, information quality, and innovation pulverization. [31]. The framework plan of BI plays out an important assignment to recover all the essential data. If there is a perspective that isn't set apart by the BI preparing and assessment gadgets, this may create an invalid record that can jeopardize the impact of the business reason. Additionally, the information limit is of incredible noteworthiness. As previously referenced, the noteworthiness of the outcomes decides the limit of data. This is, additionally, extremely imperative for prescient records. Innovation pulverization is a block in the method for finding a

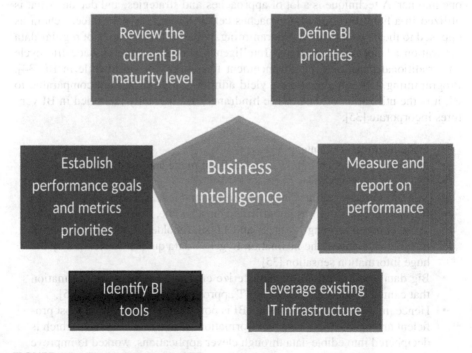

FIGURE 1.5 The business goal of BI.

workable pace and changing it. While an organization expands the amount and complexity of information, information that requires to be changed develops so huge that the equipment structure which was made five years back is currently old-fashioned. Right now, equipment framework isn't the only thing distressed by the development of a foundation. The BI framework is starting to have a blunder.

1.3.1 BUSINESS INTELLIGENCE

BI is a sort of utilization programming intended for examinations, reports, and the introduction of information that can be seen also [32]. BI programming is utilized to accomplish the procedure of appraisal, investigations, and information announcing in business [32]. Business knowledge inundates an enormous scope of approaches for automation, techniques, applications, system and machines, and the best procedure that bolsters dynamics [33]. BI is a procedure that is information-driven, and it consolidates the capacity and assortment of information with information from the board to give a contribution to the business choice procedure [33]. BI permits associations to harden the procedure of dynamics, and it includes systems, mastery, innovation, and data. BI stretches out to a general term that includes applications, apparatuses, foundation, and practices to encourage the entrance and investigation of information to upgrade execution and dynamics [34]. The challenges experienced in BI incorporate the coordinated effort of business and IT that prompts crude information turning out to be helpful data [34]. BI conveyance is done in one manner. A technique is a lot of approaches and strategies, and decides what is utilized in a field. Fruitful BI approaches center around the data esteem chain as opposed to the development of programming, which is the objective of regular data innovation advancement. Business Intelligence shows that the cascade life cycle and traditional programming advancement forms are not worthwhile in BI [34]. Programming and equipment don't yield administrative incentives comparable to BI; it is the utilization of data. Basic hindrances traditionally identified in BI ventures incorporate [35]:

- Undefined requirements.
- Inadequate reflection of how data has been made and used.
- Data quality is unknown.
- System source restraints determine design and levels of service.
- Results development was not affirmed on schedule.
- Trust is absent among business and IT shareholders. With the existence of these challenges, the inclination to get to data quicker is blended by the huge information sensation [35].
- Big data is a word used to characterize enormous compound information that cannot be solved by classical IT approaches and applications [35].
- Hence, in the scope of this article, BI is portrayed as the best and most proficient arrangement of business information from various sources, which is deciphered into edible data through clever applications, worked to improve the choices that help associations achieve their desire [35].

1.3.2 CLOUD-BASED BI MODEL

It condones various advancements that guarantee the achievement of cloud-based BI development, including distributed computing in standard cloud organization models, cloud association models, and cloud evaluating models [36]. In light of these advances, it has been comprehended that cloud BI can offer administrations through the assistance models; examples of this are, Software as a Service (SaaS), or Platform as a Service (PaaS), or Infrastructure as a Service (IaaS) in upholding in an open, private, or crossover cloud [36]. The cloud BI model is utilized in different cloud-based resources, for instance, in IaaS, to give source to frameworks and information stockpiling, and the SaaS BI application bolstered by the PaaS stage empowers business clients to customize the BI administrations given [37]. Consequently, a web-empowered condition is required for a foundation to get to BI benefits through customers [37]. Considering the consultation of the cloud-based BI model and the awareness of sensible and particular perception, a four-layer building is proposed: the presentation layer, the framework layer, the security layer, and the organization layer [37]. BI application development assets incorporate web applications, internet providers, information stockpiling, and encryption administrations. Additionally, the engineering includes specialized assets, cloud-based applications, accessibility, and security. In light of the business needs of the association, the cloud administrations can be intended to meet determined prerequisites [37].

1.3.3 CLOUD COMPUTING ROLE IN BUSINESS INTELLIGENCE

The CC in BI, however, is a kind of method that can provide adequate and safe network service [38]. Various software and hardware can be accustomed in accordance to the required customer, including server, network, storage, different software applications, services, and so on. Cloud computing has many benefits for business, and it also has difficulties [38].

1.3.4 BENEFITS AND DIFFICULTIES OF CLOUD COMPUTING IN BI

Concerning business insight in the distributed computing condition, it ought to be distinguished that distributed computing produces extraordinary open doors for BI [39]. Even though the development of distributed computing innovation is still in its beginning time, there are still such huge numbers of unsolved issues [39]. Subsequently, a few difficulties might be experienced, regardless of that, these two innovations are regularly treated to be confused advances. This can be deciphered by the way that the two innovations are presently confronting levels of popularity, most particularly their brought-together forms [39]. In this way, the absence of equipment or programming limits is essential because of lacking allotment for related undertakings. Distributed computing disperses the financial aspects of BI [40] by utilizing the equipment, system, security, and programming expected to make information stockrooms on request, on a compensation as-you-use premise. Oppositely, cloud business knowledge recommends huge dangers to the accomplishment of the business [40]. It is very sensitive to the external surroundings, in fact, and although the technology can utilize large amounts of data, it cannot be considered at first. Therefore, it mostly takes a long time to make proper expansions. Hence, this combination is not appropriate for every company in small to medium enterprises. This type of business is aligned with other critical intentions, so complicated technologies will prevent them from getting to a suitable goal range [41]. Furthermore, there is a substantial questionable significance from the context of source risk. It is quite obvious that almost half of SaaS-based applications have various effects in a cloud-based environment [41]. Concurrently, if they provide customer information with minimal boundaries, and the biggest customer-driven intelligence, the rest of the application becomes effective, which is away from the part of contemporary business data innovation. Hence, a trade-off has been accomplished on the risks and advantages of cloud business knowledge right now. Concerning any danger in enactment, it ought to be noticed that the exact moment proof of any law encroachment has been declared about the utilization of the innovation. Be that as it may, we can contend it is an extremely fitting device for an enormous scope of fabrication activity [42]. To an enormous degree, it is extremely right, however, this announcement can, without much of a stretch, be repudiated, because a few innovations are utilized for the wicked arrangement as close to home decisions, rather than the specialized and objective setting nature of cloud business insight [42]. Conflictingly, it merits saying that since cloud-based advancements adhere to the standard of everybody can see everybody, the innovation presumes little security. Consequently, any reviewing obstructions are annihilated, and the system accomplishes considerable flexibility. One of the significant elements of distributed computing is viewed as an advantage as opposed to a weakness [43]. In any case, the primary concern is to realize that distributed computing has a large stockpiling limit since it is more ensured than regular information stockrooms [43]. Consequently, operational risks are much less in a cloud-based condition. The past proclamations can likewise be determined to be as clear security benefits. Cloud-based advances need numerous layers of security, and they generally incorporate reinforcement distributed storage to ensure information, counteraction of debacles, and dangers. Effective insurance requires about a similar expense as the underlying cloud stage, so figuring is relied upon to consider its hugest parity of installments. At last, it is worth recognizing that the preparation of a worker, as a rule, longs for cost, since HR and, recently, characterized data innovation, ought to be remarkably recognized. Subsequently, this angle can't be a bit of a leeway of business insight in a cloud situation. It has made numerous foundations rebuke its utilization, regardless of whether a large portion of its points of interest and risks are decreased [43] like in Figure 1.6.

Significant advantages of source BI are:

- Improves the fulfillment of work
- Opportunity to promote new expertise
- Opportunity for the growth of the establishment
- Improvement of the status
- Eradication of endless work
- Opportunity of income management and leakages

Cloud computing in BI	
Benefits	Difficulties
• Low cost	• Internet connectivity
• Reliability	• Security limitations
• Mobility	• limited user control
• More secure	• Agreements
• More flexible	• Lower bandwidth
• Backup	• Data management
• High storage	• Technical issues
• Friendly Environment	• Limited features
• High performance	• Data mining
• Increased collaboration	• Knowledge

FIGURE 1.6 Cloud computing benefits and difficulties in BI.

1.3.5 INCORPORATING BI SOFTWARE INTO THE CLOUD

Solidifying BI into the cloud incorporating will beat the advancement oldness challenge. By so doing, adaptability it will be developed. Uniting BI into the cloud is a preferred position for an establishment for its flexibility, just as for versatility and satisfaction of use. By versatility, I raise to the furthest reaches of a BI to, as regularly as conceivable, ingest information from freshly united programming. For instance, an establishment chooses a decision at a spot that requires an online helpdesk for its clients. This can be enabled in the cloud and joined into BI frameworks in an especially specific time without the requirement for getting an extra gear, for instance, servers, to such a degree, that helpdesk programming will manage. The satisfaction of the use of a Cloud BI is picked in like manner by the straightforwardness of accessibility of BI programming on different machines. Building a web answer for helping the way toward settling on choice has the advantage of being able to associate it, whether the client remains inside the foundation or elsewhere. This will forever illuminate clients that are constantly versatile. This likewise gives responsiveness. The BI can be seen on any internet browser [34]. By utilizing stage-as-an-administration model, a BI arrangement can be empowered inside a brief period. The arrangement can take the influence of the preinstalled PaaS model, for example, similar database programming. Clients won't include in unconstrained programming the executives and piecing undertaking. The foundation of the database present on the cloud is adaptable, so it will take care of the necessities of assets plausible to lead a foundation data amount. Likewise, another advantage that is given by the cloud to BI joining is sponsored costs. Appropriating assets will exude in a decreased expense for each gadget. Likewise, equipment conservation will be overseen by the cloud supplier, just as the empowering of equipment firewalls and burden entertainers to deal with the traffic moving toward the server farm. The probability of BI arrangements is an extra benefit for associations that decide to fuse it into the cloud. By accessibility, I suggest the up time of help. Cloud structure has the capacity of working paying little mind to if the framework falls flat. Additionally, cloud suppliers ensure their web association by at least one substitute connection, so that on the off chance that one comes up short, the other will assume control over the traffic. Table 1.3 shows the points of interest and weaknesses as respects the consolidation of a BI arrangement into the cloud.

As previously referenced in the distributed computing part of this paper, security is as yet a test. BI arrangements are not excluded. The security given by BI arrangements is just at the UI organize. The information spared in the cloud database is observable to the provider. Government gauges are, in explicit cases, a square in the improvement of BI game plans of establishments to a cloud framework outside the breaking point. This symbolizes a blemish specifically of circulated registering employments. The cloud providers that are organized in a comparable country with a foundation may be costlier than outer suppliers. Cloud suppliers proffer splendidly consolidated BI arrangements that have the capacity of fulfilling a greater part of the organizations' necessities as respects BI programming. By so doing, an organization influences opening this sort of administration for outer use, like in Figure 1.7. This occasion doesn't require programming the board at all or other support matters. Any item update will be regulated by the cloud provider. There is another bit of leeway of utilizing online BI programming. Web advancement is getting increasingly more strength and customary programming programs are supplanted by online programming. An incredible advantage of web advancement is the utilization of foundations. This paces up the structure procedure of the product, and future improvement of modules is being facilitated for the made programming. Likewise, programming is dependent on the web-licensed clients to gain admittance to information nearly from any gadget just with an internet browser or a planned exceptional application.

TABLE 1.3

Advantages and Disadvantages as Regards the Incorporation of the BI Solution into the Cloud

Advantages	Disadvantages
Flexibility and scalability	Privacy
Subsidized costs	Government principles
Satisfaction of usage and access	Vendor lock-on
Cloud comparative database	Service level agreement
Availability	Legal

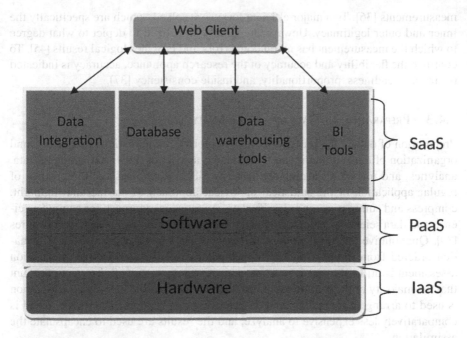

FIGURE 1.7 Basic architecture of incorporating business intelligence solutions into the cloud environment [19].

The expenses of programming are diminished by creating web innovation with BI arrangements.

1.4 PROCEDURES IN BI AND THE CLOUD

Roles in association with BI and the cloud have been efficiently used in businesses and are widely gaining popularity in modern times. These are Materials and procedures needed to produce a business intelligence system with cloud computing; they are detailed as follows.

1.4.1 COLLECTION OF DATA

The collection of data is the technique of collating and measuring information about variables of interest in a settled, orderly approach [35]. The collection of data can be chosen from different processes from various sources. BI specialists that examine and validate the expected architectural model will need to use the collected data to solve problems within establishments [35].

1.4.2 EFFECTIVENESS AND AUTHENTICITY

Solve the validity and accuracy problems to enable reliable measurement of authenticity and reliability of the measuring equipment during the process of taking measurements [36]. Two major efficient forms are solved, which are specifically the inner and outer legitimacy. Unwavering quality is utilized to depict to what degree to which the measurement has no random errors and provides logical results [45]. To continue the flexibility and accuracy of the research appliance, accuracy is indicated regarding steadiness, proportionality, and inside consistency [37].

1.4.3 Preparation of Data and Data Analysis

Preparation of data is the practice in the assemblage, combination, structuring, and organization of data so that it can be evaluated as part of the visualization of data, analytics, and machine learning applications [38]. Data analysis is the practice of regular application of the statistical or logical approach to outline and highlight, compress and summarize, and classify data. A statistical approach for computer science and data science is enforced by using data preparation and analysis procedures [39]. Quantitative data evaluation is utilized because a larger part of the information ordered from the investigation is computerized, while subjective information assessment is utilized to analyze some subjective information. Taking into account that the majority of the examined information is quantitative, factual data evaluation is used to arrange, accumulate, and descriptively display data. The data collated is comparatively less expensive to analyze, and the results are used to encapsulate the assimilation.

1.4.4 Data Surveys

Survey and evaluation has been in existence since the 1950s, and it is not a new concept [40]. The survey begins with a restricted number of sources of data from built-in systems, and the data is kept in an archive, for example, an information emporium or information storage facility, portrayed as traditional BI. Mostly analyses are quite descriptive, and BI majorly involves reports. In 2003, when high-tech companies such as Google and Yahoo started making use of big data for internal evaluation and customer-basic procedures, big data started to surface. The speed of big data changed the conventional BI because data must be gathered and prepared quickly. Predictive and normative evaluation has begun emerging, but visual analysis of detailed data remains the basic form of analysis. Big data keeps getting bigger, more plentiful, more diverse, and quicker, and establishments are beginning to concentrate on the data-steered economy. All kinds of organizations are evolving data-based products to remain competitive. With the evolvement of large information and overview, the conveyance of BI has been influenced. Information must be suddenly converted into information for evaluation. Establishments are more interested in normative and predictive evaluation that uses machine learning and rapid analysis through the process of visualization [41]. Rapid analysis can be referred to as the ability to collect and visualize data quickly. The addition in the speed of information has quickened the necessity for IT offices to catch information and convert it into helpful data.

1.5   INFORMATION TECHNOLOGY IN THE CLOUD AND BI

The IT business bloom on data and distributed computing gives the immaculate stage to testing the new programming and strategies [42]. The utilization of distributed computing is rapidly expanding, as is the data on the specialized difficulties of use. Even still, our capability of the administrative noteworthiness of distributed computing, despite everything, slacks a long way behind [43]. This overview considers the conundrum of distributed computing built up in the connection with other significant modifications in Information Technology, in which it looks at all possible progressive changes and the difficulties adhered by the specialists. After this conditional study, we investigate the meanings of distributed computing and its significant peripherals: equipment, for example, INTEL, IBM chips; administrations, for example, Google or Amazon; apps like SaaS; virtualization, for example, VMware or the blend of the segments, for instance, Citrix. At that point, we analyze the administrative centrality of distributed computing and wrap up by contending that distributed computing speaks to a significant IT change, changing how IT specialists work, in which besides a potential regulatory criticalness, there is a significant change in how administrators make an idea and oversee business [44]. Table 1.4 depicts the summary of the information technology in BI.

The survey starts by evaluating the IT pressure of unification and dissolution in line at several major stages:

- Mainframes and cluster exchange preparing, end-clients getting yields, completely brought together IT;
- PCs, end-clients processing and private business disintegration;
- Web 1.0, mass disintegration and complete association with email, home banking, web-based shopping, social communication, and so forth;
- Source of Web 1.0 plus, in which the front finish of the organization relocates to the internet, with non-intense trade preparing frameworks, and supports commoditization and being arranged at anyplace; and
- Web 2.0 in addition to distributed computing, with virtualized foundations utilizing the web 2.0 devices, net PCs, versatile innovation, and distributed computing administrations.

TABLE 1.4

Summary of Information Technology in BI

Ref	Scalability	QoS	Security	Efficiency	Performance Point
[41]	✓		✓		✓
[42]	✓	✓		✓	
[43]	✓	✓			✓
[45]		✓		✓	✓
Our research	✓	✓	✓	✓	✓

Note: QoS: Quality of Service

1.5.1   BI On-Request

BI arrangements encompassing information scouring, prescient demonstrating, and assessment are procuring importance for banks as they audit ways to deal with increment practicality while improving incomes in a profoundly forceful industry. The comprehension gotten from the reports of assessment relates to banks' capacity to put resources into a medium that gives a more noteworthy chance of ROI and are flexible to advertise requests and conduct of the clients. The ability to get to the flexible handling limit can thwart the need to configure, get, mastermind, and broaden IT systems with related costs, lead-times, and budgetary trade-off. Hence, financial establishments will take note of symbolic advantages through lower functional expenses and increase inelasticity and distribution capabilities, bringing about the realization in improved time-to-market [45].

1.5.2   Cloud Speed Up Development

Public and private clouds gives excellent simplicity to engineers to develop, update, and also test applications with financed cost and insignificant release cycles. Every association, whether little or huge, is rushed to get applications to the hands of customers quickly. Regardless, the methodology of assessment and arrangement of assets isn't being expanded at the same pace and persistently occupies an enormous measure of time. Foundations need to issue access to available, easily configurable resources to developers and testers and can bring about a reduction in cycle times and improvement in the quality of the product [46].

A compact release cycle starts with a spontaneous incorporation environment. Making use of the Right Scale Server Templates, for example, the Jenkins Template, you can discharge an unconstrained structure, test, and watching for Java, Python, and Ruby applications. The Right Scale Enterprise Edition grants you to deplete less time for the arrangement of hardware and the leading body of advantages, less time for fixing botches and redoing code, and extra time on examinations, headways, and testing. The Enterprise Edition incorporates two separate UIs: a Self-Service Portal generally worked for architects and analyzers to send servers in the cloud, and the full Right Scale Dashboard delivered for system administrators and designers to design the pre-revamped circumstances given the course of action pack [47]. The Enterprise Edition guarantees:

- On-request assets are accessible whenever they are required, making use of a self-service portal that works all over the cloud.
- Multi-Cloud Marketplace has made available the unique configurations of Server Templates, scripts, and recipes, or can be shared within your account.
- Homogeneous environments are quite easy to design and clone for testing.

1.5.3   Business Intelligence Prospects

The advantage of Business Intelligence solutions is that it helps companies to collect data or information through its three fundamental parts: joining and information extraction, information mining, and undertaking announcing frameworks. Primary significant information sources are: OLAP, which is Online Analytical Processing, the ERP, which is Enterprise Resource Planning, and CRM, which is Customer Relationship Management; these are key systems used to collect and process initial data in digital form. Business Intelligence (BI), accepted as the recent business model, has the function of connecting the breach amidst business process management and business strategy. So, it is important to examine how BI aids learning on how to deal with generalized and cumulative communications, and the maintenance of accumulative technological appliances (iPads and mobiles) that modify their features within a very minimal period. This information distributes to the governance of the projects of the establishment, such as the collective gatherings of various maintenance squads, the conveyance of the deliberation, and the job of the mediator of the deliberations projected by the squads. Especially, how effective is the business intelligence model to handle these new difficulties [48]. In the BI model, procedures enable end-users not only to view information, but also to have the technological appliances they need to comprehend the interpretation of the information separated and decide the usage to accomplish the desired outcome, whether in real-time or not. These processes request a combination and evaluation of proficiency, skills, and capabilities, as decisions are rapidly decentralized [49]. This includes scrutinizing the effect of the decentralization of the approach to information, awareness, and decision making on the performance of the people who constitute the establishment, particularly the officials. In an organizational framework that approves the permeability between the various maintenance squads, the BI model, based on the generalized response of all those included in the business venture and the exciting and proactive support in the business project, allows the discovery of what users are up to, how they go about it and where they carry it out [50]. It would be appealing to realize how the user perceives it when doing it, i.e., to interpret his feelings into data. Examining this style in the architecture of the BI model can point out if it is an important and interdependent theory.

1.6 ARTIFICIAL INTELLIGENCE (AI) IN BUSINESS INTELLIGENCE (BI)

During the era of regular stimulation of data compilation, establishments have never had this litigable acumen inside their horizon. Still, the present business intelligence approval standard lingers over 21%. However, a symbolic reason for this falter in approval is as a result of the reality that even the best business intelligence platforms stall in delivering acumen and transfer costs. And that is in speculation to if users ask the appropriate questions [51].

Nonetheless, there is a bright side; business technology is beginning to imitate the ease of usage discovered in costumer technologies in implementing artificial intelligence (AI) and machine learning (ML). We are no longer in the glorious era of customer technology. AI-based BI mechanisms expand expertise disclosure beyond the data squad and legitimize workers to reason more seriously in their duties and pull data acumen by themselves [52]. It's no wonder that companies that have approved

BI platforms in 2018 are grading product versatility, quality, and dependability at a permanent high. Below are the reasons for AI in BI implementation and the machine learning techniques used in cloud-based BI.

- **Supplies rapid responses to ad-hoc queries**
  The best time to scrutinize a query is the minute it emerges. This is not achievable with minimal business intelligence platforms that instruct data scientists to decipher the discovery, which can span up to weeks or even months to receive an answer [52]. AI business intelligence software can answer ad hoc questions accurately in a matter of moments, pulling from an organization's entire suite of data sources simultaneously.
- **Responds to questions that businesses are yet to ask**
  Probing pre-set data views and constructing routine logical reports with conventional business intelligence appliances can only help a modern establishment move forward. The automated economy grows swiftly [52]. Enterprises that cannot reason past their questions will be at loss with their competing benefits. AI-driven BI appliances move further than providing quick, precise responses to their consumer's questions; they also propose insights on questions that users did not think about! This makes the knowledge analysis procedure explorative and collective.
- **Broaden data discovery all through an establishment's network**
  The demand for data specialists is high, but they prefer, rather, to devote their time to working on complex, powerful problems that assist in the growth of the establishment in the long run. Nonetheless, most business intelligence platforms are not available enough for navigation by the average business user. This causes data squads to generate custom reports, because pre-set data views can only respond to so much [53]. This results in bottlenecks and prevents data specialists from concentrating on more challenging projects.
- **Promote outcomes, boost decision-making process, and long-term productivity**
  Text-based data leaves so much to be desired for the minor tech-savvy consumers. Even if the response appears in seconds, our brains convert images quicker than they convert text. AI in BI spontaneously combines the discovery it presents with appealing imagery [53].

  This not only enables faster data processing, but also makes sharing easy among squads and sections. AI will encourage production, whether a squad is having a deliberation and requires looking at the numbers, or a worker is making a choice in their everyday workflow.
- **AI-driven BI appliances that are transforming the industry**
  A major example of how AI-driven BI appliances are transforming the data ecosystem industry exists in features such as SpotIQ, a subsidiary of Thought Spot's data analysis platform. The motive behind SpotIQ was to construct an analysis instrument that could provide poignant business results for BI specialists and non-technical users.

SpotIQ integrates dozens of AI-powered insight-detection algorithms to capture abnormalities, trends, cross-related data, and more. These crucial elements guarantee workers do not miss important outcomes that may demand a trained eye. SpotIQ also compromises at the beginning of every discovery it presents to build up trust with the users it benefits and give them a sense of dominance in the process. In data, trust means everything. Providing clear and explainable AI that diffuse trust will be imperative to the success of smart systems [54]. The classifications of AI techniques are discussed below.

1.6.1 Supervised Learning

This is one of the most used techniques, and it is well-established. The supervised learning technique makes use of data in making exact expectations and learns the mapping between the yield and its relating input while gathering criticism through the learning procedure in distinguishing things dependent on comparative qualities. The normal methodologies completed right now are the SVM, neural systems, and relapse calculations. In preparing these calculations, for the most part, capacity is being characterized (polynomial, direct, completely associated neural system, non-linear, and so forth). This can surmise the best in connection between the yield and information. At that point, the work cost tells the understudy how far it is from the best solution. The model has the option to order business information with a precision of up to 75%. All in all, with profound learning, it has become a leap forward system right now regions.

1.6.2 Unsupervised Learning

As opposed to supervised learning that utilizes marked information, solo learning utilizes no input signal and no names. This method is ordinarily utilized in finding concealed structures of the given information and breaks it into comparative groups. It is principally utilized for descriptive demonstrating and pattern identification. This is a promising sort of computation to accomplish the general AI, yet it is lacking behind the supervised learning. Autoencoder and K-means is the most commonly known unsupervised algorithm. One of the most widely recognized employments of unsupervised learning in BI is peculiarity recognition [55]. The information created from the association will originate from comparable dispersion, and if there is any type of interruption or any bogus read from the association information, this information will be hailed an exception and can, without much of a stretch, be flagged or perceived.

1.6.3 Reinforcement Learning (Semi-Supervised)

The strategy, to a high degree, looks like how people explore and learn through their everyday schedule assignments. Reinforcement learning (RL) is neither unsupervised nor completely supervised; it is, even more, a sort of a crossbreed approach.

In RL, there is a different or single specialist that figures out how to act in a situation such that they attempt to augment their vast aggregate prize or score. At singular advances, where the present state is given, the client chooses the best activity on the reason of an approach. With this activity, the condition of nature will change, and the client gets a success sign in less than a second in the best case [56]. The client learns an optimum approach, which is the mapping from the state to activity, without going before information on nature. The arrangement is found out exclusively by experimentation, or abuse and investigation.

1.7   THE APPLICATION OF CLOUD IOT IN BATTLING COVID-19

The effect of the COVID-19 pandemic on the cloud industry has been irregular. Different cloud services and vendors have announced seeing a huge increase in rush hour gridlock [57]. The enormous scope utilization of system data transmission has been ascribed to the administrations' lockdown endeavors, which have constrained the instructive foundations to utilize online resources and organizations to permit their representatives to virtual reality. Moreover, the COVID-19 pandemic has not left the cloud area solid. Much like other cloud organizations, a lion's share of TSPs and ISPs have recorded a gigantic drop in their offer costs in recent months. The enormous scope of ramifications of the COVID-19 pandemic on the worldwide economy are ascribed to the unacceptable reaction framework received after its underlying flare-up. Even though the reaction to the COVID-19 pandemic has been more composed than the reaction to past scourges and pandemics, a couple of issues in the present pestilence/pandemic reaction framework remain [58]. These exercises are extremely applicable to other medical emergencies, as well as if there is a second/third rush of the COVID-19 pandemic later on. The cloud IoT is an amalgamation of cloud gadgets and programming applications offering broad cloud benefits that are associated with the human services IT frameworks. As of late, IoT has seen a flood in the number of its potential applications [59]. This flood is ascribed to an expanding number of cloud vendors that permit these gadgets to connect with IT frameworks [60]. Uses of cloud IoT incorporate checking patients from a remote area, following medicine requests, and utilizing wearables to transmit clinical data to the concerned clinical practitioners. Attributable to their capacity to gather, dissect, and transmit clinical information effectively, the human services area has understood the transformative capability of IoT advances [61, 62]. Amid the progress during the COVID-19 pandemic, a few trailblazers, clinical associations, and government bodies are hoping to use IoT apparatuses to lessen the weight on the social insurance frameworks. In the following, we investigate different IoT and cloud advancements that have made a significant commitment in observing, and thus, dealing with the effect of the COVID-19 pandemic.

1.7.1   MAIN APPLICATION AREA OF CLOUD IOT IN THE COVID-19 PANDEMIC

To comprehend and reduce the pandemic, numerous attempts have been published online over the recent months. Our principal intention is to show the viability of cloud intelligence to battle against the COVID-19 pandemic and survey the best arrangements utilizing these advances. Additionally, various utilizations of cloud IoT are introduced for a superior comprehension. Below, we describe various areas that utilize the cloud in battling the COVID-19 pandemic [63].

- **Quick determination and location of the disease**
  Cloud analyses can rapidly investigate sporadic side effects and other warning signs and, in this manner, alert the patients and the medical services specialists virtually [64]. It assists with giving quicker dynamics, which is financially savvy. It assists with building up another analysis and the executive's framework for COVID-19 cases through helpful virtual calculations. The cloud is useful in the finding of the COVID-19 cases with the assistance of clinical imaging advances, which enables medical analysts to communicate virtually using cloud resources.
- **Monitoring the treatment**
  Cloud IoT can enable manufacturers to create a smart stage for programmed checking and expectation of the spread of this infection. Cloud-enabled virtualization can likewise be created to remove the visual highlights of this infection. This would help in the legitimate checking and treatment of the influenced patients by giving daily updates during the pandemic [65, 66].
- **Contact follow up of the people**
  Cloud intelligence can help examine the degree of disease by this infection, distinguishing the groups and problem areas, and can effectively follow up by making contact with people and to screen them. It can anticipate the future course of this infection and likely return [67].
- **Projection of cases and mortality**
  This innovation can track and figure the idea of the infection, from the accessible information, online networking, and media stages, about the dangers of the contamination and its probable spread. Further, it can anticipate the number of positive cases in any region. Cloud-based intelligence can help recognize the most powerless locales, individuals, and nations and take timely actions [68].
- **Development of medications and immunizations**
  Cloud intelligence is used in delivering the accessible information about COVID-19. It is valuable for the medical conveyance structure and improvement. This innovation is utilized in accelerating drug testing continuously, where standard testing takes a lot of time, and henceforth assists with quickening this procedure altogether, which may not be conceivable by a human [69]. It can assist in recognizing helpful medications for the treatment of COVID-19 patients. It has become a useful asset for analytic test plans and immunization improvement remotely [70]. Cloud intelligence helps practitioners in creating antibodies and medicines at quite a bit of a quicker rate than expected, and is likewise useful for clinical preliminaries during the advancement of the immunization.

• **Reducing the burden of medical workers**

With the rapid, abrupt, and enormous increase in the quantities of patients during the COVID-19 pandemic, medicinal services experts have an exceptionally high outstanding burden. Here, cloud intelligence is utilized to lessen the outstanding task of medical services practitioners [71, 72]. It helps in early analysis and giving treatment in the early stages by utilizing advanced methodologies and virtualization. It offers the best analysis to specialists concerning this new ailment [73, 74]. Cloud intelligence can give rise to future care for patients and address increasingly potential difficulties which diminish the remaining burden of the medical practitioners.

1.8   SECURITY IN BI

The PC and IT enterprise are everlastingly tormented by criminal hackers and various security attacks; therefore, securing a business will ceaselessly be sought after. Security on distributed computing lessens the monetary costs and diminishes the additional room required on each framework [75].

1.8.1   CUSTOMER VERIFICATIONS

This is all about means of entry and who connects to the data, whether during transportation or stockpile. Routinely, associations keep their information on physical servers in their surroundings, and the equipment would require an on-location association to endanger or damage the information, which is seen to be an obstacle to hacking and illegal association [76]. Client confirmation is one of the major anxieties, even though cloud providers establish data encryption in addition to applying essential protection to track entry.

1.8.2   SAFEGUARDING DATA

No establishment would want to expose themselves to any hazard regarding their data, because the consequences of this are too huge to even envisage. Data that are frequently scrupulously restrained consists of both private and foreign data that access the establishment and customer information individually. If an establishment's security is questioned, customers will lack certainty in their services, and this will influence the general turn-over and even set the whole establishment out of business [77].

1.8.3   DATA VIOLATION, LOSS, AND DESTRUCTION

There's a significant hazard to data in cloud, especially after taking into account the different driving forces for the data exchange business. This is a security stress regardless of cloud data back-ups and different server storage facilities. To be sure, data in the cloud is less vulnerable to encroachment and physical dangers like fire, floods, etc., that are regularly a risk in physical servers [78]. Failure to grasp the entire thought of disseminated registering is, in like manner, endeavoring to be a difficulty just amidst associations wanting to use the organization for the pioneer time. That is why institutions are prune to direct anticipated security fears and =misuse..

1.8.4 STORAGE TOPOGRAPHY

You should haggle with the capacity vendor to appreciate the area of the capacity of information. This is critical for calamity arranging. For example, if a typhoon is a guideline risk to your focal data storing, and your substitute provider has its data center organized in Florida. The substitute stockpiling place ought not to be burdened by similar catastrophes [79]. You should likewise be educated of the administrative impediments in explicit organizations that may control your information from being supplied in a seaward station.

1.8.5 PUBLIC CLOUD VERSUS PRIVATE CLOUD

Although the public cloud is an adamant inclination in little organizations with fewer information stockpiling necessities, for an enormous organization, it may not reliably be an ideal inclination. This is because of the prerequisite to transmit huge amounts of information over the internet [79].

1.8.6 VERSION AWARENESS AND BACKUP EXECUTION

You should fathom how the information is put away and deciphered. In specific situations, the specialist organizations may propose just adequate reinforcements as opposed to an increasingly clever collective reinforcement arrangement. An adequate reinforcement is at both times engrossing and costly, as far as keeping up the capacity and system data transmission use [79]. On the off chance that translation is accessible, you should grasp how the understanding functions and how it very well may be joined with your information upkeep.

1.8.7 SECURITY OF DATA AND ENCODING

The data managed in the cloud must be encoded, and you should see how the encoding keys are gotten to. The specialist organization should likewise hold fast to the business determinations to create the ideal information security. When selecting the service provider, make time to comprehend their service-level agreement and ensure it follows your specifications. You should become familiar with the information and the foreseen time to re-establish the opportunity substances [79].

1.9 POTENTIAL HAZARDS OF CLOUD BI ADOPTION

Similarly, the potential dangers of cloud Business Intelligence appropriation ought to be apprehended. The study is especially disturbed with the hazards concerned in the acceptance procedure. For instance, the most extensive approval of risk is about selecting the most suitable pricing model. One of the subsequent consulting schemes will focus on this matter in data analysis [80]. The above risks are very common, since they have made many establishments take delicate approaches to enhance their critical arrangement. Potential hazards of cloud BI in adaptation are:

- Absence of approving assets
- Shortage of cloud understanding
- Resizing in departments
- Mistrust in new evolving technology
- Rise independence on foreign mediators
- Reduction in work satisfaction

1.9.1 SECURITY DIFFICULTIES

In distributed computing, clients don't have a clue about the specific purpose of their sensitive information, since cloud specialist organizations hold server farms in topographically separate areas, which leads to various security troubles and dangers [80]. Ordinary security advancements like firewalls have antivirus programming, and interruption revelation frameworks don't give satisfactory security in virtual frameworks because of the fast spread of dangers inside virtual conditions [80].

1.9.2 THREATS AND RISKS IN CLOUD COMPUTING

Below, we highlight twelve security threats in common cloud BI [79]. Out of every one of these dangers, information ruptures are pinpointed as the most significant security issue to talk about.

- Data breaches (crack)
- Jeopardized credentials and damaged certification
- Hacked interface and Application Program Interfaces (API)
- Abuse of cloud services
- Account hijacking
- Malignant associates
- Advanced Persistent Threat (APT) parasite
- Abused system vulnerabilities
- Permanent loss of data
- Diligence inadequacy
- Attacks by Denial of Service (DoS)
- Shared technology, shared dangers

1.9.3 PRIVACY AND SECURITY

Data privacy is very crucial, and it is one of the core issues limiting users' trust in any business [81]. Implicit authentication mechanisms and privacy protection are what the application must support to keep data secure and gain users' trust in the cloud system [81]. In providing what is said to be a secure connection or communication over a network, an important player is the encryption algorithm. In the protection of data, it is a fundamental and valuable tool. Using the encryption algorithm, the data is converted and scrambled in a form, and a "key" is used just particularly for the user to decrypt the data. Symmetric key encryption is an important technique that researchers have researched [81]. Only one key is used in encrypting and decrypting data in symmetric key encryption.

1.10 DISCUSSION AND OPEN RESEARCH

In designing a cloud business intelligence system in cloud computing, the architecture and methodology have to be discussed. Also, the significance of using business intelligence and the background in association with cloud computing has to be discussed. The authors have proposed concentrations on the evolution of cloud computing in business intelligence systems. Research issues are open, including the various information assessment strategies and the necessities of distributed computing and the issue of security for the protection of information. In light of the genuine issues in distributed computing, security troubles and business rules which are in connection with innovation are as yet an open issue for analysts.

Online Analytical Processing, or OLAP, is the core or the main technology used in many business intelligence applications. Predicting a what-if scenario, planning (forecasting, budget), calculating complex analysis, including viewing unlimited reports, and discovery of data are some of the powerful technology OLAP can provide.

Today, data analytics has been an eye-opener for so many companies; BI in the cloud is providing solutions to problems and is becoming a common area in enterprises. Quality of accurate data-driven insights is needed more than ever by businesses. To the community of business users, a primary interface is being implemented by SaaS. BI functionality as a service is a concept initiated by cloud BI. DELETE, INSERT, UPDATE, are part of the online short transactions characterized by OLTP.

The amount of transactions per second in the measure of effectiveness and the integrity of data being maintained across multiple environments is a very fast process of query that OLTP focuses on. On the other hand, low transaction volumes are relatively characterized by OLAP. Queries involve aggregation and are majorly very complex. The measure of effectiveness is referred to have the response time in OLAP systems.

Besides, internet communication is a very critical issue in high-speed cloud computing. The existing technologies in close area computing networks are working fine, but when we talk about cloud computing in wide area networks, a fast connection must be ensured. Usually, high-speed internet connections in wide area networks consume a huge amount of energy, resulting in escalating computing costs. Therefore, low-energy efficient networks must be developed to ensure quality communication in cloud computing.

1.11 CONCLUSION

Cloud computing, for certain years now, is represented to be the prominent innovation as respects adaptability and flexibility. Utilizing shared assets gives an extraordinary advantage to a creating organization. This is likewise reflected in consumptions. Not exhausting a great deal into equipment infrastructures and its administration will empower the organization to grow a lot quicker by expanding into development, showcasing, and so on. Joining BI programming in the cloud enveloping is critical if the affiliation intends to achieve a bit of leeway. The historical backdrop of business insight is given in detail to absorb what the significant standards of business knowledge are. The BI model design situated in the cloud and the obligation of cloud computing are disclosed in subtleties to find out about the cloud BI structure. The advantages and difficulties are likewise depicted with regards to the utilization of distributed computing. This arrangement will introduce an organization to the significant devices to confront its rivals. The satisfaction of utilization and approach that a cloud BI proffers will enable the laborers to have versatility without changing the system of dynamics. Some future research that should be carried out with regards to BI, is that business and technology continues to grow in age and time. Be that as it may, the central enthusiasm of utilizing a BI arrangement in the cloud encompassing is comparable to protection. This test will continue until a feasible game plan is reached. This arrangement may be the encryption programming that can settle in the cloud. The BI model had the option to order business information with a precision of up to 75%. All in all, with profound learning, it has become a leap forward system right now in regions.

ACKNOWLEDGMENTS

We give all praise to almighty Allah for the success of this paper. Also, we would like to acknowledge Prof. Dr. Fadi Al-Turjman for his support and contributions to the successful completion of this paper.

REFERENCES

1. Zahmatkesh, H., and F. Al-Turjman. (2020). Fog computing for sustainable smart cities in the IoT Era: Caching techniques and enabling technologies - an overview. *Elsevier Sustainable Cities and Societies*, 59, 102139.
2. Al-Turjman, F., and C. Altrjman. (2020) Enhanced medium access for traffic management in smart-cities' vehicular-cloud. *IEEE Intelligent Transportation Systems Magazine*. DOI. 10.1109/MITS.2019.2962144.
3. Baars, H., and H.-G. Kemper. (2010). Business intelligence in the cloud. Paper presented at the Pacific Asia Conference on Information Systems (PACIS).
4. Reyes, E. P. (2010). *A Systems Thinking Approach to Business Intelligence Solutions Based on Cloud Computing*. Massachusetts Institute of Technology.
5. Thompson, W. J., and J. S. Van der Walt. (2010). Business intelligence in the cloud. *South African Journal of Information Management*, 12(1), 1–15.
6. Armbrust, M., A. Fox, R. Griffith, A. D. Joseph, R. Katz, A. Konwinski, and M. Zaharia. (2010). A view of cloud computing. *Communications of the ACM*, 53(4), 50–58.

7. F. Al-Turjman. (2020). Intelligence and security in Big 5G-oriented IoNT: An overview. *Elsevier Future Generation Computer Systems*, 102(1), 357–368. (**IF 5.76**).

8. Baars, H., and H.-G. Kemper. (2008). Management support with structured and unstructured data: An integrated business intelligence framework. *Information Systems Management*, 25(2), 132–148.

9. Moss, L. T., and S. Atre. (2003). *Business Intelligence Roadmap: The Complete Project Lifecycle for Decision-Support Applications*. Pearson Education.

10. Kimball, R., and M. Ross. (2002). *The Data Warehouse Toolkit: The Complete Guide to Dimensional Modeling* (2nd ed.). New York: Wiley.

11. McKnight, W. (2007). Moving business intelligence to the operational world, part 1. *Information Management*, 17(8), 28.

12. Mohammed, A. B., J. Altmann, and J. Hwang. (2010). Cloud computing value chains: Understanding businesses and value creation in the cloud. In *Economic Models and Algorithms for Distributed Systems*, D. Neumann, M. Baker, J. Altmann and O. Rana (Eds.) (pp. 187–208). Birkhäuser Basel.

13. McKnight, W. (2007). New age data warehousing. *DM REVIEW*, 17(11), 49.

14. Vaquero, L. M, L. Rodero-Merino, J. Caceres, and M. Lindner. (2008). A break in the clouds: Towards a cloud definition. *ACM SIGCOMM Computer Communication Review*, 39(1), 50–55.

15. Hayes, B. (2008). Cloud computing. *Communications of the ACM*, 51(7), 9–11.

16. Al-Turjman, F., and S. Alturjman. (2018). Context-sensitive Access in Industrial Internet of Things (IIoT) Healthcare Applications. *IEEE Transactions on Industrial Informatics*, 14(6), 2736–2744.

17. Mell, P., and T. Grance. (2009). *The NIST Definition of Cloud Computing*. National Institute of Science and Technology.

18. Cloud computing and medicine [Online]. Available: http://www.xinn.com/cloud computing-and-medicine/.

19. Rodero-Merino, L., L. M. Vaquero, V. Gil, F. Galán, J. Fontán, R. S. Montero, and I. M. Llorente. (2010). From infrastructure delivery to service management in clouds. *Future Generation Computer Systems*, 26(8), 1226–1240.

20. Cloud computing and saas information technology evolving [Online]. Available: http://www.cloudtweaks.com/2012/02/cloud-computing-and-saasinformation-technology-evolving/.

21. Educational institutions and cloud computing: A roadmap of responsibilities [Online]. Available: http://www.huffingtonpost.com/danieljsolove/educationalinstitutions_b_2156612.Html.

22. Youseff, L., M. Butrico, and D. Da Silva. (2008). Toward a unified ontology of cloud computing. Paper presented at the Grid Computing Environments Workshop, GCE '08.

23. Van Haren Publishing. (2007). *It Service Management: An Introduction*. Van Haran Publishing.

24. Winniford, M. A., S. Conger, and L. Erickson-Harris. (2009). Confusion in the ranks: IT service management practice and terminology. *Information Systems Management*, 26(2), 153–163.

25. Above the clouds: A view of cloud computing [Online]. Available: http://mars.ing.unimo.it/didattica/ingss/Lec SaS/CloudView.pdf.

26. Kern, T., M. C. Lacity, and L. Willcocks. (2002). Net Sourcing: Renting Business Applications and Services Over a Network. FT Press.

27. Chaudhry, S., H. Alhakami, A. Baz, and F. Al-Turjman. (2020). Securing demand response management: A certificate based authentication scheme for smart grid access control. *IEEE Access*, 8(1), 101235–101243.

28. Al-Aqrabi, H., L. Liu, R. Hill, and N. Antonopoulos. (2015). Cloud BI: Future of business intelligence in the Cloud. *Journal of Computer and System Sciences*, 81(1), 85–96.
29. Alsufyani, R., and V. Chang. (2015). Risk analysis of business intelligence in cloud computing. In IEEE 7th International Conference on Cloud Computing Technology and Science (Cloud Com). IEEE.
30. Salih, Q., M. Arafaturrahman, F. Al-Turjman, and Z. Rizal. (2020). Smart routing management framework exploiting dynamic data resources of cross-layer design and machine learning approaches for mobile cognitive radio networks: A survey. *IEEE Access*, 8(1), 67835–67867.
31. Bauer, E. (2018). Cloud automation and economic efficiency. *IEEE Cloud Computing*, 5(2), 26–32.
32. Bellini, P., D. Cenni, and P. Nesi. (2015). A knowledge base driven solution for smart cloud management. IEEE 8th International Conference on Cloud Computing. IEEE.
33. Chang, V., Y. Kuo, and M. Ramachandran. (2016). Cloud computing adoption framework: A security framework for business clouds. *Future Generation Computer Systems*, 57, 24–41.
34. Al-Aqrabi, H., L. Liu, R. Hill, and N. Antonopoulos. (2015). Cloud BI: Future of business intelligence in the cloud. *Journal of Computer and System Sciences*, 81(1), 85–96.
35. Kim, Y., and E. Huh. (2017). Towards the design of a system and a workflow model for medical big data processing in the hybrid cloud. In IEEE 15th Intl Conf on Dependable, Autonomic and Secure Computing, 15th Intl Confon Pervasive Intelligence and Computing, 3rd Intl Conf on Big Data Intelligence and Computing and Cyber Science and Technology Congress (DASC/PiCom/DataCom/CyberSciTech). IEEE.
36. Larson, D., and V. Chang. (2016). A review and future direction of agile, business intelligence, analytics and data science. *International Journal of Information Management*, 36(5), 700–710.
37. Liang, T., and Y. Liu. (2018). Research landscape of business intelligence and big data analytics: A bibliometrics study. *Expert Systems with Applications*, 111, 2–10.
38. Sahmim, S., and H. Gharsellaoui. (2017). Privacy and security in internet-based computing: Cloud computing, Internet of Things, Cloud of Things: A review. *Procedia Computer Science*, 112, 1516–1522.
39. Stergiou, C., K. Psannis, B. Gupta, and Y. Ishibashi. (2018). Security, privacy & efficiency of sustainable cloud computing for big data & IoT. *Sustainable Computing: Informatics and Systems*, 19, 174–184.
40. Stergiou, C., K. Psannis, B. Kim, and B. Gupta. (2018). Secure integration of IoT and cloud computing. *Future Generation Computer Systems*, 78, 964–975.
41. Subramanian, N., and A. Jeyaraj. (2018). Recent security challenges in cloud computing. *Computers & Electrical Engineering*, 71, 28–42.
42. Sekaran, R., R. Patan, A. Raveendran, F. Al-Turjman, M. Ramachandran, and L. Mostarda. (2020). Survival study on blockchain based 6G-enabled mobile edge Computation for IoT automation. *IEEE Access*, 8(1), 143453–143463.
43. Al-Turjman, F., and S. Alturjman. (2018). 5G/IoT-enabled UAVs for multimedia delivery in industry-oriented applications. *Springer's Multimedia Tools and Applications Journal*. DOI: 10.1007/s11042-018-6288-7.
44. Thompson, W.J. J, and J. S. van der Walt. (2010). Business intelligence in the cloud. *South African Journal of Information Management*, 12(1),1–5.
45. Review study: Business intelligence concepts and approaches, [Online]. Available: http://www.researchgate.net/profile/Vahid_Mirhosseini/publication/256667827 Review:Study_Business_Intelligence_Concepts_and_Approaches/links/00b7d5239641b7b653000000.pdf.

46. A model for business intelligence systems' development, [Online]. Available: http://rev istaie.ase.ro/content/52/10%20-%20Bara,%20Botha.pdf.
47. The cloud computing: The future of BI in the cloud, [Online]. Available: http://www.ijct e.org/papers/404-G1093.pdf.
48. A systems thinking approach to business intelligence solutions based on cloud computing, [Online]. Available: https://www.google.ro/url?sa=t&rct=j&q=&esrc=s&sou rce=web&cd=10cad=rja&uact=8&ved=0CFwQFjAJ&url=http%3A%2F%2Fdspace. mit.edu%2Fbitstream%2Fhandle%2F1721.1%2F59267%2F667715636.pdf&ei=VOUF VY3NFcLuaJzZgqgF&usg=AFQjCNGNbQ106ZK5v6337ClWEDOFUizPlQ&sig= F2lvDePELe5vWNtTpfXrqQ.
49. Industries that will gain from adopting the cloud, [Online]. Available: http://www.clou dtweaks.com/2012/09/10-industries-that-will-gainfrom-adopting-the-cloud/.
50. Creating your cloud based backup and data recovery strategy [Online]. Available: http: //www.cloudtweaks.com/2012/03/creating-your-cloud-basedbackup-and-data-reco very-strategy/.
51. Kern, T., M. C. Lacity, L. Willcocks. (2002). *Net Sourcing: Renting Business Applications and Services Over a Network*. FT Press.
52. Educational Institutions, [Online]. Available: http://www.huffingtonpost.com/daniel-j-solove/educationalinstitutions_b_2156612html.
53. Fenn, J., and H. LeHong. (2011). *Hype Cycle for Emerging Technologies*. Gartner.
54. How mobile cloud computing is set to change the telecommunications ecosystem, [Online]. Available: http://www.cloudtweaks.com/2012/09/how-mobile-cloudcomp uting-is-set-to-change-the-telecommunications-ecosystem/.
55. Al-Turjman, F., M. Z. Hasan, and H. Al-Rizzo. (2019). Task scheduling in cloud-based survivability applications using swarm optimization in IoT. *Transactions on Emerging Telecommunications,* 30(8). DOI: 10.1002/ett.3539.
56. Al-Turjman, F. (2019). Intelligence and security in big 5G-oriented IoNT: An overview. *Elsevier Future Generation Computer Systems*, 102, 357–368.
57. Deloitte. Understanding COVID-19's impact on the telecom sector. Accessed: [Online]. Available:https://www2.deloitte.com/global/en/pages/about-deloitte/articles/covid% 19/understanding-covid-19-impact-on-the-telecom-sector.html, (2020).
58. Sohrabi, C., Z. Alsafi, N. O'Neill, M. Khan, A. Kerwan, A. Al-Jabir, C. Iosifidis, and R. Agha. (2020). World health organization declares global emergency: A review of the 2019 novel coronavirus (COVID-19). International Journal of Surgery, 76, 71–76.
59. Hassija, V., V. Chamola, V. Saxena, D. Jain, P. Goyal, and B. Sikdar. (2019). A survey on IoT security: Application areas, security threats, and solution architectures *IEEE Access*, 7, 82721–82743.
60. Rouse, M. (2015). What is IoMT (Internet of Medical Things) or healthcare IoT. [Online]. Available: https://internetofthingsagenda.techtarget.com/definition/IoMT-Int ernet-%of-Medical-Things.
61. Deloitte Centre for Health Solutions. Medtech Internet Med. Things. [Online]. Available: https://www2.deloitte.com/content/dam/Deloitte/global/Documents/Life-S c%iences-Health-Care/gx-lshcmedtech-iomt-brochure.pdf, (2018).
62. Rodrigues, J. J. P. C., D. B. D. R. Segundo, H. A. Junqueira, M. H. Sabino, R. M. Prince, J. Al-Muhtadi, and V. H. C. De Albuquerque. (2018). Enabling technologies for the Internet of health things. *IEEE Access*, 6, 13129–13141.
63. Ai, T., Z. Yang, H. Hou, C. Zhan, C. Chen, W. Lv, Q. Tao, Z. Sun, and L. Xia. (2020). Correlation of chest CT and RT-PCR testing in coronavirus disease 2019 (COVID-19) in China: A report of 1014 cases. *Radiology*. [Online]. Available: https://doi.org/10.1 148/radiol.2020200642.

64. Kolhar, M., F. Al-Turjman, A. Alameen, and M. Abualhaj. (2020). A three layered decentralized IoT biometric architecture for city lockdown during COVID-19 outbreak. *IEEE Access*. DOI: 10.1109/ACCESS.2020.3021983.
65. Al-Turjman, F., and D. Deebak. (2020). Privacy-aware energy-efficient framework using internet of medical things for COVID-19. *IEEE Internet of Things Magazine*. DOI: 10.1109/IOTM.0001.2000123.
66. Rahman, M., N. Zaman, A. Asyharia, F. Al-Turjman, M. Bhuiyan, and M. Zolkipli. (2020). Data-driven dynamic clustering framework for mitigating the adverse economic impact of Covid-19 lockdown practices. *Elsevier Sustainable Cities and Societies*, 62, 102372.
67. Stebbing, J., A. Phelan, I. Griffin, C. Tucker, O. Oechsle, D. Smith and P. Richardson. (2020). COVID-19: Combining antiviral and anti-inflammatory treatments. *The Lancet Infectious Diseases*, 20(4), 400–402.
68. Hussain, A., O. Bouachir, F. Al-Turjman, and M. Aloqaily. (2020). AI techniques for COVID-19. *IEEE Access*. DOI: 10.1109/ACCESS.2020.3007939.
69. Waheed, A., M. Goyal, D. Gupta, A. Khanna, F. Al-Turjman, and P. R. Pinheiro. (2020). CovidGAN: Data augmentation using auxiliary classifier GAN for improved Covid-19 detection. *IEEE Access*. DOI. 10.1109/ACCESS.2020.2994762.
70. Bobdey, S. and S. Ray. (2020). Going viraleCOVID-19 impact assessment: A perspective beyond clinical practice. *Journal of Marine Medical Society*, 22(1): 9.
71. Ozsoz, M., A. Ibrahim, S. Serte, F. Al-Turjman, and P. Yakoi. (2020). Viral and bacterial pneumonia detection using artificial intelligence in the Era of COVID-19. *Research Square*. DOI: 10.21203/rs.3.rs-70158/v1i.
72. Pirouz, B., S. ShaffieeHaghshenas, S. ShaffieeHaghshenas, and P. Piro. (2020). Investigating a serious challenge in the sustainable development process: Analysis of confirmed cases of COVID-19 (new type of coronavirus) through a binary classification using artificial intelligence and regression analysis. *Sustainability*, 12(6): 2427.
73. Gupta, R., and A. Misra. (2020). Contentious issues and evolving concepts in the clinical presentation and management of patients with COVID-19 infection with reference to use of therapeutic and other drugs used in Co-morbid diseases (Hypertension, diabetes etc.). *Diabetes & Metabolic Syndrome: Clinical Research & Reviews*, 14(3): 251e4.
74. Gupta, R., A. Ghosh, A. K. Singh, and A. Misra. Clinical considerations for patients with diabetes in times of COVID-19 epidemic. *Diabetes & Metabolic Syndrome: Clinical Research & Reviews*, 14(3): 211e2, (2020).
75. Al-Turjman, F., and D. Deebak. (2020). Smart mutual authentication protocol for cloud based medical healthcare systems using internet of medical things. *IEEE Journal on Selected Areas in Communications*. DOI. 10.1109/JSAC.2020.3020599.
76. Krafzig, D., K. Banke, and D. Slama. (2005). *Enterprise SOA: Service Oriented Architecture Best Practices*. Prentice Hall Professional Technical Reference.
77. Al-Turjman, F., and D. Deebak. (2020). A novel community-based trust aware recommender systems for big data cloud service networks. *Elsevier Sustainable Cities and Societies*, 61. DOI: 10.1016/j.scs.2020.102274.
78. Wang, L., J. Tao, M. Kunze, A. C Castellanos, D. Kramer, and W. Karl. (2008). Scientific cloud computing: Early definition and experience. Paper presented at the 10th IEEE International Conference on High Performance Computing and Communications, HPCC '08. IEEE.
79. Ibrahim, U., M. Ozsos, and F. Al-Turjman. (2020). Futuristic CRISPR-based biosensing in the Cloud and Internet of Things Era: An Overview. *Multimedia Tools and Applications*. DOI: 10.1007/s11042-020-09010-5.

80. Cloud computing security and trust workshop, [Online]. Available: http://labs.safelaye r.com/en/research-and-development/focusareas/security-trust-and-privacy/460-clou d-computing-securityand-trust-workshop.
81. Papazoglou, M. P.(2003). Service-oriented computing: Concepts, characteristics and directions. Paper presented at the Proceedings of the 4th International Conference on Web Information Systems Engineering (WISE). IEEE.

2 Resource Allocation in Volunteered Cloud Computing and Battling COVID-19

Adedoyin A. Hussain and Fadi Al-Turjman

CONTENTS

2.1   INTRODUCTION

Cloud volunteer computing provides computing services that manage applications and statistics by using the internet and secluded central servers, for a fee. Volunteers don't gather monetary profits for their resource; however, they may get open regard as computation winnings [1]. Computations carried out with volunteer computing sometimes represent global issues, such as predicting the climate [1] or the discovery of drugs for cancer. This idea permits clients and also businesses to make use of applications without putting their information at any PC having internet access.

This thought likewise takes into consideration considerably more capable computing by concentrating stockpiling, service model, virtualization, and bandwidth. Some examples based on the models of cloud computing are Gmail, Google app engine, Dropbox, Hotmail, etc. Cloud computing operates more like a help instead of a product, whereby shared assets, programming, and data are given to PCs and other methodologies. Cloud computing gives access on-request to virtual assets like systems, servers, stockpiling, middles and application, and administrations [2]. These resources can quickly be provisioned and give little administration exertion or no communication from the specialist organization [2]. Volunteer computing clouds particular volunteered resources from the broad public to implement computations. It is coordinated around common criteria, be it digital, by tools sharing between many single teams carrying out research, or physically, by making volunteers add their computing resources to a large number of projects.

Resource allocation is the way toward assigning assets accessible to the customers as indicated by their needs. It is also the assigning of resources available to cloud applications that need them over the internet [3]. The major intent of the cloud resource providers and clients is to assign cloud resources proficiently and accomplish the most noteworthy money-related benefit. Cloud computing proposes various algorithms that are used in allocating resources. Data centers make use of these algorithms in utilizing different virtual machines on servers. The algorithms are Bin Packing [4], Priority algorithm [4], Bees [5], and ACO (Ant Colony Optimization) [6]. For efficient resource allocation, these algorithms can be implemented.

- Ant Colony Optimization algorithm: the ACO implements an ant's behavioral approach for food collecting. In this approach, ants merge in a group in search of the collection of food in an efficient way that is good for them.
- Bees algorithm: Bees algorithm is based on how bees collect their food. In contrast to the ant algorithm, jobs with the lowest memory are found by a meta-scheduler.
- Priority algorithm: Priority Algorithm is a dynamic allocation of resources for jobs that are preempted able in the cloud, while the allocation of resources is performed following their requirement.
- Bin Packing algorithm: this algorithm depends on the reason for pressing items of a particular weight into a given limit of bins.

From the client's line of sight, allocating resources refers to how resources and services are circulated into the midst of clients. The efficiency of allocating resources results in a more industrious economy. The clients hardly use the resources they need for a fastidious job when deploying skills as a service; this eliminates making payment for computing resources that are unused by the client. Price investment can go ahead in resource allocation where clients are being permitted to make use of current software and contribute to the environment to promote business modernization, but this is not so when it comes to volunteered computing. It diminishes the physical equipment and programming requests from the client's side [7]. The main thing expected to run by the client is the cloud chipped in registering framework interface programming, which can be as straightforward as a Web program, and the Cloud arrangement deals with the rest. We, as a whole, have encountered cloud chipped in processing assets at some moment; a portion of the well-known cloud administrations we have utilized, or we are as yet utilizing, are mail administrations like Gmail, Hotmail, or Yahoo, and so on. Resources from cloud volunteered computing equips little businesses with constrained resources successfully; it gives independent ventures access to the advancements that beforehand were out of their range; the assets encourage private companies to develop and also converts their maintenance cost into more profit.

There are a lot of territories for the use of resource allotment in cloud volunteer computing. Different endeavors have been made on planning calculation dependent on the portion of assets. High throughput, greatest proficiency, Quality of Service (QoS) aware, most extreme vitality and force utilization, and so forth, are parameters that are being considered in asset designation in the cloud. In the accompanying section a brisk audit of the resources in cloud volunteered computing will be discussed. Also, the essential features associated with the cloud will be discussed in Table 2.1.

2.1.1 Comparison to Other Surveys

The heterogeneous system is referred to as cloud computing due to the fact that it holds different and huge types of data in a large amount. However, these days, due to the growth factor of technology, cloud volunteer computing is a developing process

---

TABLE 2.1
Essential Features of Cloud Resources

Features	Goal
Easy-to-use Services	These resources are requested on-demand; with this, users demand services over the internet; they make use of the available resource as a metered service [8]. These resources are used following customers' requirements, thus bypassing resource wastage.
Simple Network Access	The simplicity of the internet is an additional advantage; accessing the internet requires a device and an internet connection. Also, with the use of a browser, users request these volunteered resources from the cloud [8].
Resource Constructiveness	Most times it is said to be the concept of cloud resource because it breaks down one physical gadget into at least one virtual gadget, which users request on demand [9].
Flexibility and Elasticity	This is an important aspect for its ability to dynamically scale down or up, and fluctuation of traffic and request from users [9].
Available Services	Small businesses and large enterprises can also benefit from these resources dynamically. With this, they pay for only the resource that is being used which is cost-effective [10].

in innovation technology. In this way, in using the resources in the cloud, processing costs must be decreased, the performance of servers must be increased, and processing and completion time must also be minimized; it is also necessary to schedule a cloud task for efficiency, whereas volunteered computing gets this recourse voluntarily. So, the major objective is the allocation of the tasks or resources in the cloud. Several authors have proposed several allocations of resource algorithms to solve the problems associated with it. This paper [11–13] discusses in detail about cloud computing and volunteered computing. Fundamentals and various applications associated with cloud computing and volunteered computing are discussed by the authors of these papers. There are works for the analysis of resource allocation in the cloud. Several scheduling algorithms for allocation of resource have been discussed and attempted. Numerous parameters are to be considered concerning resource allocation in the cloud, like high throughput, efficiency at its pick, SLA, QoS, maximum energy, etc. [13, 14], which are some reviews done on resource allocation in the cloud. There has been a couple of surveys carried out concerning the scheduling of resources. For example, in Ref. [15], the authors have slightly touched on the concept, with the main focus on the differences in types of scheduling. In paper [16], the author discusses more about the processing of data in the cloud. An open-source programming model was introduced. MapReduce is said to be a programming model that supports implementation in processing and managing large data. MapReduce model is easy to use; even users that are new to the cloud and lack experience in distributed or parallel systems do not need to worry, since parallelization, locality optimization, fault tolerance, and load balancing are hidden [16]. Countless issues of various kinds can easily be expressed by computation in MapReduce. In [17], the author implemented the development of MapReduce; it scales up cluster machines which consist of many machines in their thousands. Several things were found from [17]. The programming model is restricted in a way for distributed computations and parallelization to become easy, making use of computation fault-tolerant and redundant execution in reducing the effect of moderate machines and taking care of disappointments in machines and loss of information. Concerning security issues and attacks, a comprehensive categorization and a promising solution has also been discussed. Moreover, we have shed some light on open research areas such as communication and authentication mechanisms, the development of reliable means to assure security, and also paving a way for the future and new technology, since the cloud is an emerging field. A summary of some works in resource allocation is discussed in Table 2.2.

2.1.2 Scope of the Paper and Contributions

The examples mentioned above are areas where resource allocation and services have made great achievements. Concerning the studies mentioned, for the efficient use of new allocation paradigms introduced to the cloud, it is important to explore and comprehend the difficulties related to the idea of the cloud and resources. Right now, we will show a preview for resource allocation and emphasize certain procedures

TABLE 2.2

Comparison to Other Surveys

Reference	Power	Reliability	QoS	Security	ML	Cost	Efficiency
[5]		✓		✓		✓	✓
[6]	✓	✓	✓	✓	✓		✓
[7]	✓		✓	✓	✓		✓
[8]	✓		✓	✓	✓		✓
[9]	✓		✓	✓	✓		✓
[10]		✓	✓	✓		✓	✓
[13]	✓	✓	✓	✓		✓	✓
[14]		✓	✓	✓	✓		✓
[18]		✓	✓	✓		✓	✓
[19]		✓	✓	✓	✓		✓
[20]	✓	✓	✓		✓		✓
Our survey	✓	✓	✓	✓	✓	✓	✓

and strategies to be kept in thought while managing difficulties. In like manner, our principle contribution in this work can be outlined as follows:

- This survey provides an overview of the volunteered resources over the cloud.
- We summarize and outline security measures and requirements.
- Expected and common security threats are overviewed and discussed.
- We outline the potential artificial intelligence in volunteer cloud resource management techniques.
- We categorize different machine learning (ML) techniques.
- We summarize the associated scheduling techniques and their design factors.
- We outline the main roles of the associated entities in the cloud.
- Finally, open research challenges and issues are discussed.

This paper is sorted out as follows. We overview, in Section 2.2, the role any entity plays in the cloud, in association with resource allocation. In Section 2.3 we discuss, in-depth, the resources in cloud volunteer computing, including intelligence and MapReduce. In Section 2.4, we discuss the scheduling of resources in the cloud. Algorithms of resource allocation are discussed in Section 2.5. In Section 2.6, we discuss cloud and IoT in COVID-19. In Section 2.7, we talk in-depth about the security of the resources and the security issues and challenges respectively. In Section 2.8, we outline the open research and discussion about resource allocation in the cloud. Finally, Section 2.9 is the conclusion on our thoughts and contribution, which we have introduced in this survey. For more understanding and readable information, Table 2.3 provides a summarization of the abbreviations used in addition to their definition.

TABLE 2.3
The List of Used Abbreviations

Term	Abbreviation
ABC	Activity-Based Costing
BAR	Balance-Reduce
BS	Balanced Spiral
COA	Course of Action
DAG	Directed Acyclic Graph
DPSA	Dynamic Priority Scheduling Algorithm
DRR	Deadline Reliability Resources-Aware
IaaS	Infrastructure as a Service
IoT	Internet of Things
IP	Internet Protocol
LAN	Local Area Network
MAGA	Multi-Agent Genetic Algorithm
NAS	Network Attached Storage
QASA	QoS–Aware Scheduling Algorithm
QoS	Quality of Service
RL	Reinforcement Learning
SaaS	Software as a Service
SAN	Storage Area Network
TCP	Transfer Control Protocol
TUF	Time Utility Functions

2.2 ROLES OF ANY ENTITY IN THE CLOUD

Entities in the cloud play a special role in the cloud, which involves the delivery of cloud computing or cloud volunteered computing. This sets up equipment and programming relegated by a cloud provider, who conventionally works or intercedes for a cloud integrator. It, for the most part, includes various cloud assets speaking with one another over an application interfaces, typically a web administration. A block diagram of the role of the entities is illustrated in Figure 2.1, and it will be discussed in detail below.

2.2.1 PROVIDER

Cloud resource providers manage and operate computing systems live on the cloud to provide services and resources to clients or third parties. Required expenditure, billing, and management create a higher barrier to entry, which significantly creates an overhead [21]. Moreover, even smaller organizations realize efficiency in significant operations and advantages in agility; even rollouts in virtualization and server consolidation is well underway.

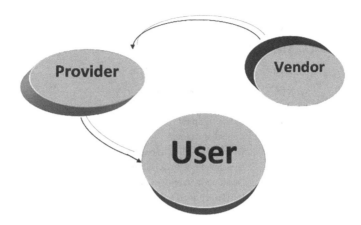

FIGURE 2.1   Entity Roles in the cloud.

Places like Amazon are said to be one of the first providers, with modernized data centers and optimizing 10% of its ability anytime, leaving a space for spikes occasionally, just like most computer networks. This facilitates fast-moving small groups in adding new features faster and easier, and ends up opening it to outsiders as a utility computing basis, like Amazon Web Services in 2002 [22].

2.2.2   USER

A client is just the shopper of cloud volunteer processing or distributed computing assets. Protection in the cloud is a significant worry among clients. Sellers have taken a stab at providing an answer by forming productive security into their administrations, for example, encryption and confirmation [23]. Clients' rights are additionally an issue; making a bill of rights is being sought after by the network to address this issue.

With virtualization, it offers a versatile arrangement of much independent smart gadgets; inert processing assets can be allotted and utilized all the more effectively, in which the client finds a good pace. Virtualization gives the quickness expected to accelerate IT activities and limits cost by expanding the use of foundation. The point of a cloud asset is to make clients gain from these innovations, dismissing the prerequisite for profound information about or proficiency of either of them [22].

2.2.3   VENDOR

All aspects that facilitate the delivery, adoption and the use of cloud tools are sold by the vendor as products and services. Examples are computer hardware (HP, Sun Microsystems), storages (EMC, IBM), infrastructures like computer programming resembles, operating frameworks, and platform virtualization; all these companies provide resources to the users [24].

The vendor also works on improving the agility for its organizations, as cloud volunteer computing increases users' flexibility, and also on re-provisioning, adding, or broadening technological frame-work resources. Cloud applications do not require installation on each user's computer, but can be reached from different places that are being maintained by the vendor.

2.3 RESOURCES IN CLOUD VOLUNTEER COMPUTING

Cloud volunteer computing provides a reasonable computing architecture for online businesses, clients, and projects in which they make use of these resources on-demand, for free. In Table 2.4, we summarize the work done in allocating these resources.

2.3.1 STORAGE-BASED RESOURCE

Cloud storage is a service model resource rendered by the vendor to the client in which data is aggregated, handled, backed up, and made available to a client remotely over a network. Cloud data storage used by the client is paid on a monthly rate per-consumption, but will be free since it is volunteered. Nevertheless, the cost although radically been driven down per gigabyte, eliminating the cost of large physical storage. Moreover, operating expenses have been added by the storage vendor that make the technology more expensive than expected by the client [26]. Security in clouds is a major concern among users. Vendors have tried creating a solution by developing efficient security into their services, such as encryption and authentication [27]. Cloud backup, recovery, and archiving infrequently accessed data are some of the most commonly used cases of storage in cloud volunteer computing. A larger number of clients make use of cloud storage services for development options, which serves as a capital measure for cost-cutting. They can call on any storage resource at any time, depending on the duration of the project at hand. Listed are some areas of storage in the cloud.

2.3.1.1 Network Storage

Network storage is used in describing, usually, a large number of devices sectored together which are available over a network. Storages like this maintain copies, at high-speed, of data across a LAN connection and are to back up records, databases, and other information to be gathered in a focal area, so it tends to be effectively gotten to through standard system conventions and instruments. There are two fundamental standard kinds of system stockpiling, which are known as a) Storage Area Network (SAN) and b) Network Attached Storage (NAS). Business systems, using very good quality servers, high-limit circle clusters, and fiber channel interconnection innovation, are essentially utilized by SAN. NAS is related to the Home system, which introduces equipment named NAS gadgets onto the LAN through TCP/IP. Table 2.5 gives a detailed distinction between these two types of network storage.

TABLE 2.4
Summary of the Works in Resource Allocation

Author and Ref	Algorithm	Environment	Goal	Year
Xue et al [19]	Multi-Target Genetic	Cloud	• The cost of resources has been reduced. • Balancing of loads.	2014
Salimi et al [20]	Multi-Target Genetic	Grid	• The cost of resources has been reduced. • Balancing of loads.	2014
Cheng [21]	Genetic	Cloud	• Time for the longest termination time has been reduced. • Balancing of loads.	2012
Gomathi & Karthikey [25]	Swarm Optimization	Cloud	• Time for the longest termination time has been reduced. • Balancing of loads.	2013
Pandey et al [21]	Swarm Optimization	Cloud	• Load balancing cost has been reduced.	2010
Wu et al [22]	Swarm Optimization	Grid	• Workflow time has been reduced. • Balancing loads.	2012
Izakian et al [23]	Swarm Optimization	Cloud	• Time for the longest termination time has been reduced. • Workflow time has been reduced. • Balancing of loads.	2010
Banerjee et al [24]	Ant Colony	Cloud	• Time for the longest termination time has been reduced. • Balancing of loads.	2009
Mousavi & Fazekas [26]	Ant Colony	Cloud	• Time for the longest termination time has been reduced. • Workflow time has been reduced. • Balancing of loads.	2016
Moallem [27] CloudSim	Ant Colony	Grid	• Time for the longest termination time has been reduced. • Balancing of loads.	2011
Babu & Krishna [28]	Bee Colony	Cloud	• Time for the longest termination time has been reduced. • Balancing of loads.	2013
Zhao [29]	Swarm Optimization	Cloud	• Time for the longest termination time has been reduced. • Resources cost has been reduced.	2015
Abdullah & Othman [30]	Simulated Annealing	Cloud	• Time for the longest termination time has been reduced. • Balancing loads.	2014

TABLE 2.5
The Differences between NAS and SAN

	NAS	SAN
Fabric	TCP/IP network is used and, commonly, Ethernet.	Works on high-speed fiber channel.
Data processing	File-based data processing.	Block data is being processed.
Protocols	Ethernet network is connected directly. NFS, SMB/CIFS, and HTTP are various protocols in connecting to the server.	SCSI protocol is used in communication with the server.
Performance	Bags the advantages of higher latency and lower throughput due to the file system layer being slow.	Requires higher speed traffic for higher performance in the environment.
Scalability	They are highly scalable, even up to petabytes making use of clusters.	The major driver is its scalability. Performance and capacity are being scaled due to network architecture.
Ease of management	Management is easy. A simplified management interface is being offered by NAS.	More administration time is required than NAS.
Price	It is less expensive to maintain and purchase, although high-end NAS will cost more.	It is more complex to manage.

2.3.1.2 Hard Disk

The hard disk is one of the main resources, and usually large in partitioning, data are also being stored. On the hard disk software titles, the operating system and most other files are stored. All these are made virtually available to the client. IaaS (infrastructure as a service) is a type of the mill administration model; to cause the framework to fortify, virtual volumes of incessant provisioning, and brief provisioning is required. However, the performance of the hard disk drive storage might not be sufficient, and this can lead to a bottleneck. Some examples are solid-state drive (SSD), normal HDD storage, and distributed storages [31]. The hybrid model achieves a much higher performance in contrast to the normal HDD storage; with this advantage, it is efficient in analyzing applications. The performance of the distributed storage in degradation is lower in contrast to the normal HDD storage when the number of concurrent processes is being increased and is suitable in archiving a large number of files for storage.

2.3.2 NETWORK-BASED RESOURCE

Organizations host their networking resources on the cloud; this is known as cloud networking, and this is made possible by the cloud vendor. It may be referring to the public or private cloud. Computing resources are centralized and are shared between users; this scenario is made possible based on cloud resources. Networks are being shared in the same way, and this has spiked a trend in implementing more network-related functions into the cloud environment. Table 2.6 provides differences and goals between each trend.

2.3.2.1   Reliable Communications
This improves late commitment between resource allocation and adaptation to non-critical failure, which tradeoff in asset imperative framework later on. The frequent request of gigabit Ethernet has given growth in acceleration to investigate an enhancement in producing a 400 gigabit per second Ethernet standard. Looking forward, there has been a consensus of producing, eventually, a 1 Tbps.

2.3.2.2   Efficient Communications
A congestion exposure process was proposed by IETF to achieve congestion proportionality for network resources, sharing computation, and storage. Moreover, this issue is still opened for discussion. This will enable efficient communication between users.

2.3.2.3   Virtual Networking
Several authors have proposed the future evolution of virtualization in the cloud network, where cloud-based web applications are being predicted and the paradigm of the client sever becomes absolute. Peer to peer, developing a collaborative and a pervasive web environment was envisioned for the fate of the web in cloud-based web applications. Other aspects are also being visited for the efficiency of virtualization in networking.

2.3.3   SERVICE MODEL AS A RESOURCE
The service model provides computing or IT as an assistant over a system or web as a metered administration on-demand, based on how it is being used, but users get

TABLE 2.6
Networking Trends in Cloud Computing

Computing Main Area	Goal
Strong communications	This upgrades the Gigabit Ethernet between resource distribution and adaptation to non-critical failure making answers for exchange of.
Efficient communications	This is creating an efficient way of sharing cloud resources among tenants in a federated cloud system, making communication efficient to users.
Virtual networking	Peer to peer, developing a collaborative and a pervasive web environment is to be studied for the customer server worldview to get out of date.
Other pressing areas	Network virtualization functions, IoT, computing architectures for inter-Cloud.

the advantage of no pay when it is volunteered. The service ranges from servers to development platforms, applications, virtual desktops, and storage. Government and private bodies utilize cloud services like data storage and database, and compute in addressing some application and infrastructure needs. The architecture of the service models is illustrated in Figure 2.2 below. These cloud services are being delivered in minutes to hours, and costs are aligned to actual usage. Due to consumer's utilization of resources like storage, sharing, and accessibility from any web-connected device, the organization has higher agility in managing more expenses efficiently. Table 2.7 talks about attributes associated with the service models below.

2.3.3.1 Infrastructure as a Service (IaaS)

These are basic computer tools like storage, networking, etc. These are made available to users in the form of virtualization instance with the use of virtual technology. Operating systems and applications are owned and managed by the user over a metered service.

2.3.3.2 Software as a Service (IaaS)

These are applications running on the website. The software, which is provided to the user over the internet is managed and owned by the SaaS provider. This software is accessed as a metered service over a yearly or monthly subscription. Examples are Dropbox, Gmail, etc.

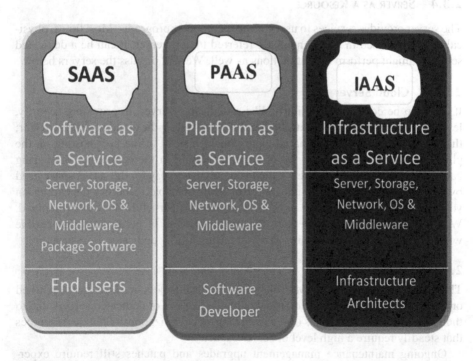

FIGURE 2.2   Service model.

TABLE 2.7

Common Attributes Associated with Cloud Computing Services

Attribute	Explanation
Virtualization	Allocation and reallocation of resources for server and storage virtualization are being utilized rapidly by cloud computing.
Multi-tenancy	By gaining economies of scaled resources are being shared and pooled admits multiple users.
Network accessibility	Web-browser or thin client access resource using different types of networked devices.
On-demand	Resources from the online catalog of pre-defined configurations are self-provisioned.
Elasticity	Resource can scale quickly and effortlessly.
Metering/chargeback	Resource usages are a metered service based on service arrangement.

2.3.3.3   Platform as a Service (PaaS)

These are software provided to developers to build their cloud application by PaaS provider. Users make use of this scheme as a metered operation.

2.3.4   SERVER AS A RESOURCE

The server provides services to users or other computer programs. Most times, physical computers used in data centers are referred to as a server. It can be a dedicated server or might perform other functions as well. We will discuss the servers below.

2.3.4.1   Cloud Server

It can also be configured similarly, like a dedicated server, in providing security, levels of performance, and controls. But this is hosted by the cloud hosting provider; they reside in a virtualized shared environment instead of the user hosting on the physical hardware. There is a lot of benefit, ranging in the economics of sharing hardware with various customers which you only get to pay for the server space used by the user. You will get the advantage of using scalable resources depending on your demand, so you won't be paying for an idle infrastructure due to low demand. With the advantage of cloud servers, the optimization of IT performance is possible without the fear of cost managing and purchasing a fully dedicated infrastructure.

2.3.4.2   Dedicated Server

This is simply a dedicated server solely for a user's business needs, either purchased or rented. Large businesses and organizations make use of dedicated servers due to their exceptionally high levels of securing data, or organizations of data or resources that steadily require a high level of server capacity.

Ongoing maintenance management upgrades and patches still require expertise and IT capacity for businesses using dedicated servers. Dedicated bare-metal hardware provides significant value for big data platforms and databases for businesses making use of I/O-heavy applications.

2.3.5 MapReduce AS A RESOURCE

Map-reduce provides an efficient way for organizations that produce a large quantity of data. The large data set is therefore divided into smaller data chunks and therefore shared among application processing components. The results are individually consolidated later. These lead to how efficient large amounts of data are being handled by cloud applications. The scalability of distributed applications gives advantages for the distribution of data processing amidst multiple application component instances in a similar manner. Hence, the important aspect is the frameworks and parallel algorithms, which is the ability in processing a large volume of data and meeting performance requirements entailed for such data analyses. MapReduce has been proven efficient in that area and has gained large popularity in the aspect of a resource in data analysis. The programming model of MapReduce as a calculation that takes a group of (key, value) combines as input and produces a (key, value) matches as output [29]. MapReduce library, as used by the user, states the process as two functions (Mappers and Reducers). A little arrangement of potential values is shaped by blending the qualities gotten from the reduced function written by the user as a set of values for that key, called an intermediate key. The mapping process maps the value in order to produce the intermediate key as its output. The whole process of moving from the mappers to the reducers is called the shuffling process.

Hadoop application is just an open-source execution for MapReduce. It utilizes MapReduce as an explanatory motor while in the engine, utilizing an appropriated circulated capacity layer alluded to as Hadoop distributed file system (HDFS). In Hadoop distributed file system, the entire local disk is being mapped into a single file hierarchy system, enabling the spreading of the data across other nodes. Throughput of jobs in Hadoop is a big challenge due to the local processing of data, this can be overcome by enhancing the efficiency of the locality by assigning data to corresponding nodes [32]. However, there must be a slot available for computing for processing a task with the corresponding data with computing nodes, so when a schedule is done for the task, the locality is improved. For instance, when a slot is not available, the task must be rescheduled to a remote node. In reacting to each VM in a virtual cluster for various demands, there must be a dynamical reconfiguration for each VM. However, there is no availability for the dynamic reconfiguration of VM currently in cloud services. Figure 2.3 shows the illustration of the MapReduce scheme.

2.3.6 INTELLIGENCE AND RESOURCE ALLOCATION

The resource allocation scheme is implemented by allocating services between users and service providers; it is optimized best on a different scale at the point when a savvy approach is being executed. It is a typical perspective in any asset administration to watch crafted by AI (Artificial Intelligence) and generally ML

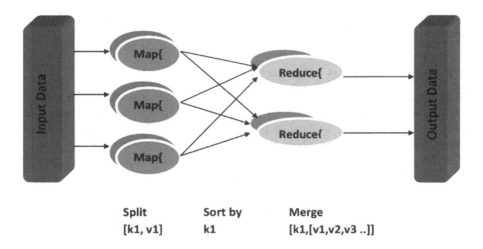

Split	Sort by	Merge
[k1, v1]	k1	[k1,[v1,v2,v3 ..]]

FIGURE 2.3 MapReduce layout.

(machine learning) procedures, while giving a simple way of life to clients to propel the straightforwardness of the resource use. Aside from the fact that ML is being used to optimize and manage the operation of resource usage, it also has an advantage in understanding and finding insight on collected data [25]. For example, ML is implemented in health care systems in understanding the kind of disease associated with each patient; this actually enhances the health care monitoring board system and also helps in predicting the future of an outbreak. Some of the issues associated with intelligence in ML are discussed in Table 2.8. The order of ML methods falls into three classifications. The classification depends principally on the sort of information and the target of the data in association with the resource. They are as follows:

2.3.6.1 Supervised Learning

This is the common technique used, and it is well established. It makes an accurate prediction by feeding on data, and it learns how to map between the input and the corresponding output of that data while receiving feedback on the learning process in correlating and identifying things based on a pattern or features that are similar. Classifying of input into desirable classes and outcome prediction are associated to this category [33]. The neural network, regression algorithms, and support vector machine (SVM) are common approaches associated with this category. In introducing the training associated with these techniques, normally a function that approximates the best between output and input is defined. They can be polynomial, non-linear, fully connected NN, or linear, etc. The cost function then tells the learner how far it can be from the best answer, which means it goes about as a criticism. Then the feedback is used in updating the parameters of the function at each iteration. Finally, in predicting input of the future or classification of the unseen data, this function will be used.

TABLE 2.8

Issues Associated with Intelligence in ML

Design Issue	Description
Data Redundancy and Duplication	This means at least the same value is being represented by more than one data instance.
	Using pairwise similarity comparison techniques problems are being created by redundancy, but not adding value.
Data Noise	This is part of a data indicated for cleaning due to incorrect and missing values. Noise is being created by outliers and data sparsely in ML models.
Data Heterogeneity	These are the different data formats and files, data type samples amongst variables.
Data Discretization	This occurs when converting quantitative to qualitative data. Decision trees and Naïve Bayes are some algorithms that require this process.
Data Labeling	Semi-supervised, supervised, active, and transfer learning require this method.
Feature Selection	This is when data properties are identified, and its influential effect is more. In feature engineering and feature selection, a prior knowledge domain is needed, and feature selection requires intensive labor.

2.3.6.2 Unsupervised Learning

In contrast to supervised learning, which utilizes information being labeled, unsupervised learning utilizes no marked information and no criticism. Finding structures hidden in data and moving it to a similar group is mostly associated with this category. Descriptive modeling and pattern recognition are what this category is mainly used for. In achieving general AI, these algorithms are promising; usually, they lack accuracy, and delay is another factor, unlike the supervised learning. Some popular algorithms for unsupervised learning are K-means and autoencoder [18].

2.3.6.3 Reinforcement Learning (Semi-Supervised)

The method in which humans learn their everyday life tasks, to a high extent, resembles this technique. It is an approach of a hybrid model because it is not fully unsupervised or supervised. With this, it gathers both advantages. Resource data are to be processed and generated at most instantly. Advanced adaptive algorithms are used in addressing key challenges for this learning technique, like structural data change [34]. Typically, most times are spent on preprocessing and understanding the data; also, another timing factor is deploying and developing learning techniques. At the training stage, the efficiency of the learning technique can be reached by the availability of valuable and usable data.

2.4   SCHEDULING OF RESOURCES IN THE CLOUD

Resource scheduling in volunteered computing is a critical procedure, as it incorporates countless information among clients and the volunteered resource. Keeping up this information assumes a vital job in improving usage and limiting the finish and reaction time of these assets [35]. Considering all these, scheduling is an unquestionable requirement [36]. The engineering of the scheduling scheme is portrayed in Figure 2.4. The scheduling scheme, in association with the priority level, rate of arrival, and the dedicated server, is being updated frequently, as depicted in Figure 2.3. However, the scheduling scheme updates frequently, including the number of committed servers for each class in understanding their need level and appearance rate. Parallelism capabilities require many complex applications. Scheduling of resources must be done correctly, so there will be an increase in response time within resources as well, to avoid a decrease in completion time. Some types of task scheduling will be discussed as follows.

2.4.1 CLOUD SERVICE SCHEDULING

Cloud administration scheduling is classified as client and system level. At the user level, issues are handled between providers and customers about resource provisioning, while the system level relates to the management of resources within the data center [20].

In the data center, a large number of physical machines are present. Tasks of over a million, from users, are received; these tasks are assigned at the data center to each physical machine. The data center performances are impacted by this scheduling or assignment [37]. Some facts to be taken into consideration for system utilization are

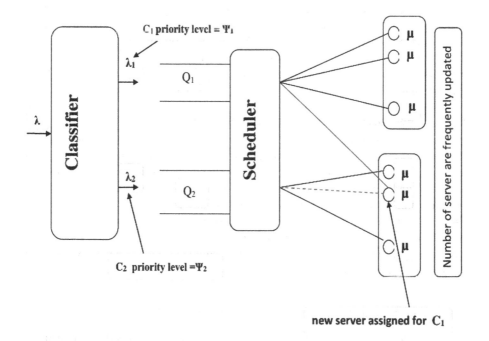

FIGURE 2.4 Architecture of the scheduling scheme.

resource sharing, adaptation to non-critical failure, SLA, dependability, continuous fulfillment, QoS, and so forth.

2.4.2 CUSTOMER SIDE SCHEDULING

In controlling resources and their demands, customer side scheduling can be categorized as auction- and market-based at the user level. The user's request for the resource is dynamic, which it scales up and down in demand for resources; because of this, a market-based allocation of resources was proposed. IaaS implements this mechanism. Auction-based scheduling is implemented by service providers as a virtual machine type [37].

2.4.3 STATIC AND DYNAMIC SCHEDULING

Static scheduling permits users to get details of the data in advance. This data will undergo a pipelining concept in parallel processing, reducing the runtime. In dynamic scheduling, execution time is specified to the server distribution of assignments and is done on the fly [38].

In different stages of task execution in data and pipelining, prefetching is allowed in static scheduling. Runtime overhead is lessened in static scheduling. Job components/tasks for dynamic scheduling information is not known beforehand. Flextic is an environment for job execution that provides a flexible pricing model for the user by using a scalable static scheduling technique at the same time and reduces overhead for scheduling for the service-giver, as in [39]. Resource providers, specialist co-ops, and customers are in three levels of administration demand; planning systems in cloud structure are to fulfill the shoppers and the specialist organizations. As proposed, dynamic needs booking calculation (DPSA) in [40] to gain the objective as above. MaxRe is a fault-tolerant scheduling algorithm, like in [41]. A powerful number of reproductions for various tasks are being exploited by this algorithm into the active replication schema, which also incorporates the reliability analysis. Scheduling model is a trust mechanism-based task as proposed in [42]. A Bayesian cognitive method is being scored by utilization and by the trustworthiness of nodes, and among computing nodes, a trust relationship is built. A job scheduling mechanism for feedback dynamic algorithm was proposed by authors in [42]. For the situation where resource contentions are fierce for utilization of resources in cloud volunteered computing, feedback preemptible scheduling is used in improving it. Measuring the expense of cloud assets precisely is impossible by the conventional path for task scheduling in cloud volunteered computing, the reason being that they are the total difference between cloud system tasks. An optimized algorithm is introduced, as in [43], for scheduling of activities for ABC (activity-based costing) in the cloud. Hybrid cloud environments for dynamic scheduling with different optimization experiment strategies are performed as proposed in [43]. Backfill algorithm method utilizes the adjusted winding (BS) technique to achieve QoS in the cloud environment, as proposed in [44]. EASY, conservative, and CBA various parallel scheduling job algorithms are analyzed in this paper. DRR scheduling algorithm considers the correspondence model and reasonable system topology as in [44]. Reinforcement learning (RL) is proposed [45] for recuperation situations in the cloud substances, considering the failure and recovery while maximizing utilities and making job scheduling fault-tolerable in the long term.

2.4.4 HEURISTIC SCHEDULING

Optimization problems make use of this scheduling scheme. NP-hard problems are used in classifying this. Optimization solution is used for this kind of problem. Enumeration, approximation, or heuristic methods are scheduling algorithms used for this purpose [46]. An optimal solution in the enumeration method is selected by comparison of each solution one by one; an increase in several solutions decreases the effectiveness of the enumeration algorithm. In finding suboptimal solutions, heuristic scheduling is used to produce reasonable response times quickly [46].

In finding an optimized solution for approximate solutions, an approximation algorithm is required. When we know the exact polynomial-time algorithms, this algorithm is used for such problems associated with it. The job completion time is crucial in large-scale data processing systems for enhancing task data locally. Ignoring global optimization and being greedy are issues concerning approaches in improving data locality. Balance-reduce (BAR) was proposed in addressing a heuristic task scheduling algorithm problem, as in [47]. While trying to minimize the task set span, the entire system load is balanced by the heap adjusting task scheduler. Balancing technique for cloud loading [47], in cloud environment utilizes its capacity to balance dynamic mechanism. In deciding to outsource a workload to a service provider, utilization of the internal infrastructure is to be maximized, and the cost of running should be minimized while noting the quality of service constraints of applications. In a multi-cloud environment, a scheduling algorithm for multi-objective meta-heuristics is proposed [48]. While diminishing the application cost and keeping the heap resource, amplifying the calculation, achieves high availability of application and fault-tolerance. In scheduling independent and divisible tasks, an optimized algorithm based on GA to adapt to different memory requirements and computation is proposed in [48]. Solving the load balancing problem, a hybrid algorithm of GA called multi-agent genetic algorithm is proposed [49]. Allocating resources and also scheduling involves a COA plan. Various time planning for a robust COA on GA is mentioned in [49]. Distribution of geographical location, heterogeneity, administrative constraints, energy consumption, and transparency are used in identifying the computing system scalability.

2.4.5 WORKFLOW SCHEDULING

Directed Acyclic Graph (DAG) is used in considering this scheduling as an application. Implementing the DAG of tasks, every individual node is considered as a solution to the tasks available for the user's problem, and inter-task dependencies represent edges as in [50]. They will be communicated within the task in the workflow. A directed acyclic graph form is a way of structuring of applications enabled by workflow [50] where a constituent task is represented by each node, and inter-task dependencies for application are represented by edges [51]. Communication may occur between each set of tasks and another task in the workflow; this generally implies a single workflow. Management of workflow execution is one of the key factors in Workflow scheduling. An environment of workflow scheduling algorithms survey is presented in [51]. Scheduling algorithm types and issues, including various problems for cloud workflow, is studied in [52]. Cloud workflows of instance-intensive study is proposed in [52].

2.4.6 REAL-TIME SCHEDULING

A decrease in normal reaction time and increment in throughput is one of the primary objectives of this scheduling [53]. In cases where there is a need for QoS, real-time scheduling is applied, which is known as QoS–aware scheduling algorithm (QASA). Minimizing average response time and increasing throughputs are one of the core objectives of real-time scheduling. Non-preemptive scheduling of real-time tasks was proposed with the main goal of utilizing maximization to the fullest [53]. A profit and penalty TUF are the two types of utility function; these are associated at some time with each task. The early completion of the stated approach is not just rewarded, but also gives a penalty to the aborted task or real-time tasks deadline. The preemptive algorithm is similarly imposed in [54]. An approach of real-time driven workload is proposed in [54]. Signal data processing guarantees QoS for some applications is an important area. SAQA is a QoS-aware scheduling algorithm that is self-adaptive [54], QoS demands on heterogeneous clusters to consider adaptability for real-time tasks.

2.4.7 DYNAMIC DEDICATED SERVER SCHEDULING (DDSS)

The use of cloud computing has expanded additional time over the customary strategies because of the simplicity of upkeep, straightforwardness of utilization, time and vitality productivity, paying more only as costs arise, and flexibility of data access [55]. Long unwanted delay and decrease in throughput in the scheduling of cloud servers can be due to the inefficiency of the cloud server. This DDSS can further be sub-classed into homogeneous and heterogeneous [55]. Heterogeneous server means the rate of service for all servers can as well be different, because a failed or misbehavior of a server of a multiple server system is being replaced by powerful or more new ones, which make the system heterogeneous [16]. Therefore, while considering building architecture in cloud volunteered computing, a heterogeneous server should be considered. The slowest server first (SSF) and fasted server first (FSF) give rise to heterogeneity in the distribution of services to the customers. A homogeneous server means the rate of service for all servers is equivalent when contrasted with the past homogenous DSS planning. However, it is wise to compare performance analysis between the homogeneous and heterogeneous using the slowest server first (SSF) and fasted server first (FSF) [56]. Authors have compared the performance of the utilization of DDSS against two typical building architecture that is to be considered for server scheduling, namely slowest server first (SSF) and fasted server first (FSF), while varying the utilization as shown in Figure 2.6, which also shows the utilization of DDSS, h-DDSS, and SSF, FSF in contrast to Figure 2.7. If it is worth saying, C1 increases in priority level over C2, which reduces in utilization while utilization improves in C2 of DDSS. However, with the drop rate for h-DDSS, the classes are gotten through an analytical model and simulation. The drop rate in C2 increases with time for both simulation and analytical models, and C2 decreases, which makes C2 higher than C1, as shown in Figures 2.5 and 2.6. Figures 2.7 shows an illustration of throughput respectively for h-DDSS; the classes are gotten through analytical models and simulation. Both simulation and analytical models match. The drop rate in C1 is higher than that of C2, like in [56]. However, there is equality in rates of service over all servers. In Table 2.9 is the list of notations used.

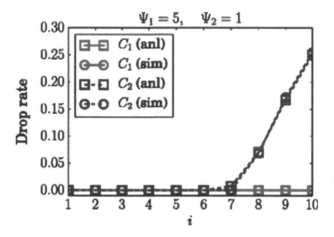

FIGURE 2.5 H-DDSS (FSF allocation) drop rate gotten through an analytical model and simulations [56].

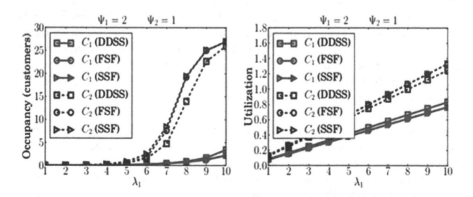

FIGURE 2.6 DDSS and h-DDSS classes being utilized with SSF and FSF [56].

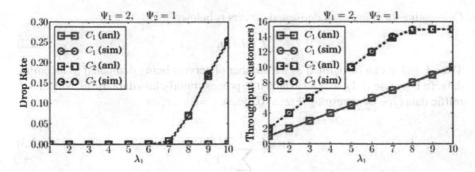

FIGURE 2.7 Throughput of classes for DDSS and hDDSS with SSF and FSF [56].

TABLE 2.9

Notations Used

Notations	Quantity
Pi	Probability of I number of C1 users in the framework.
Λ	Rate of arrival for users.
λ_1, λ_2	Rate of arrival of C_1 and C_2 users.
Ψ_1, Ψ_2	Priority level of C_1 and C_2 users.
μ_i, η_i	Service initial rate of dedicated i servers for C_1 and C_2 users.
μ_{ti}, η_{ti}	Total service rate of dedicated servers for C_1 and C_2 users until the ith server.
μ_{total}	System total service rates.
m, k	The specific number of servers for C_1 and C_2.
N	Size of Q_1.
Δ	Queue average delay of C_1 users.
N	Queue average occupancy of C_1 users.
D	Drop probability of C_1 users.
Γ	Throughput of C_1 users.

These are a few conditions concerning a few parameters allotted to every data traffic class and additionally for every application mentioned. The errand of the DDSS booking is abridged in portraying the quantity of offered servers to classes of every data traffic, and updating is done routinely dependent on Equations (2.1) and (2.3) below, as in [57]. One of the points of the necessary booking of DDSS [57] is the capacity to allocate diverse server gatherings to particular solicitations' classes, dependent on Equation (2.1):

$$\frac{I\Psi_1\lambda_1}{\sum_{t=1}^{n}\Psi_1\lambda_1} \tag{2.1}$$

Calculating the number of dedicated servers is below:

$$k = l - m, \tag{2.2}$$

Thus, k and m can be defined as the number of servers being dedicated to incoming data. In Equation (2.1), we can extend it to process multi-class data traffic with an "r" traffic data type by assuming $\Psi_\iota \lambda_\iota \neq 0$, where $\iota = \{1,\ldots,r\}$ as

$$\mu_{tm} = \frac{\mu_{\text{total}} \Psi_\iota \lambda_1}{\sum_{l=1}^{r} \Psi_l \lambda_1} \tag{2.3}$$

The authors proposed an algorithm in Ref. [28] considering three essential parameters that empower a powerful scheduling: (i) the paces of arrival for C1 and C2 customers ($\lambda 1$, $\lambda 2$), (ii) the levels of priority for C1 and C2 customers ($\Psi 1$, $\Psi 2$), and (iii) the rate of the all-out assistance in the framework (μtotal). These three parameters can be utilized to infer all-out help rates (μ_{tm} and ηtk) allotted to each class of clients, as in Equations (2.1) and (2.3). Indeed, μ_{tm} is a perfect complete help rate allocated to C1. In any case, it is hard to accomplish the equivalent whole of heterogeneous pace of administration to μtm. Accordingly, the quicker servers (aggregate of servers of these servers are around equivalent to μtm) are doled out to the higher need class.

2.5 ALGORITHMS OF RESOURCE ALLOCATION

Resource allocation is just a procedure of dispensing resources to the customers or clients as per their needs. Different calculations are being used for asset designation in the cloud chipped in registering. For the capability of asset assignment in the cloud, these calculations can be executed. In booking virtual machines on servers at various servers, these calculations are focal points for that task. ACO (Ant Colony Optimization), Bees, Bin Packing, and Priority are the algorithms. These algorithms will be discussed below. Resource allocation algorithms:

2.5.1 ANT COLONY OPTIMIZATION ALGORITHM

ACO is simply ants' conduct when drawing closer or gathering nourishment. Right now, ants make frames in bunches looking for and gathering nourishment dependably and effectively for them [58]. The essential standard identified with the algorithm is the conduct and disposition of the ant while moving between sources, for example, a goal to settle (nourishment), or the other way around. The algorithm firstly checks if there is an available resource, then a set of optimal nodes is selected after some factors are analyzed, like response time. Then the job is allocated to the suitable nodes [59]. Figure 2.8 shows an image of the ant algorithm.

2.5.2 BEES ALGORITHM

This technique is based on how bees get their nourishment. Right now, in this aspect, in contrast to the ant algorithm, jobs with the lowest memory, processor requirement,

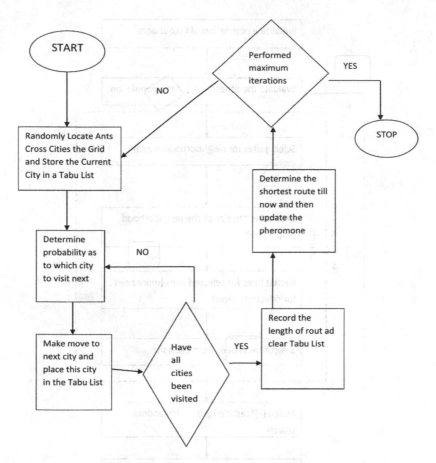

FIGURE 2.8 A Flow-Chart representing the AOC algorithm [58].

and input-output are found by a meta-scheduler [30]. This job acts in the form of a scout bee in finding a suitable or appropriate site. The job being scouted is sent to a location in which the task is needed by the resource at present. The location is identified by the scouting job making use of a fitness function. At a particular instance, the fitness function runs the task and then evaluates the task to know whether it is processor dependent or memory dependent. The progress of an assigned resource with a particular job is called fitness. After the location and resource are identified, the scouting job returns to meta-scheduler and then the waggle function is performed. Segregation of the task present in meta-scheduler is done by the waggle function on the premise of the given data by jobs being scouted, for example, memory necessities, cost, and processor [30]. Figure 2.9 shows a flow chart of this algorithm.

2.5.3 PRIORITY ALGORITHM

Priority algorithm is dynamic resource allocation idea for jobs that are preemptable in the cloud; this is the allotment of assets for clients in understanding their necessity,

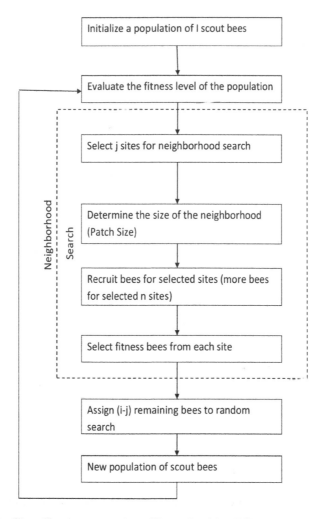

FIGURE 2.9   Flow Chart representation of Bees algorithm [30].

and Cloud min-min scheduling algorithm is lesser in performance compared to the priority-based scheduling algorithm [60]. When the cloud scheduler receives a job in priority algorithm, it will be divided into the task in the understanding of their conditions, and afterward, the algorithm is called to shape a rundown of assignments in agreement with their priority level. The list of virtual machines and available resources is forms which task can be allotted to. The appropriate virtual machine and resources are decided by the algorithm, and then it is allocated to the task on the list [60].

2.5.4   BIN-PACKING ALGORITHM

Bin packing is based on pressing objects of a given size into a given limit of containers. The one-dimensional bin, the size identified with each article, is the genuine

TABLE 2.10

Algorithm Factors

Reference	Energy	QoS	ML	Cloud Environment	Evolutionary Algorithm
[58]		✓	✓	✓	✓
[30]	✓		✓	✓	✓
[60]		✓	✓	✓	✓
[61]	✓		✓	✓	✓
Our research	✓	✓	✓	✓	✓

number that is somewhere in the range of 0 and 1, and the receptacle size is the same, given that the sum of all the objects in the bin should not be more than 1. Best fit algorithms in the cloud are used by the bin-packing algorithm. Bin size, weights, and a given list of objects, utilizing these, it then looks for the smallest amount of bin for the cumulative of the assets which are then allocated to that specific bin [61] (Table 2.10).

2.6 USAGE OF CLOUD AND IOT IN COVID-19

COVID-19 has pushed a greater part of the IT industry to embrace the work-from-home model. IT and cloud ventures have empowered a portable workforce, embracing undertaking portability instruments and administrations. Along these lines, there is an expanded interest for cloud correspondence and coordinated effort benefits over the globe. Cloud is assisting with handling catastrophe recuperation circumstances utilizing appropriated cloud IT frameworks. Inferable from the absence of an on-location IT workforce amid the lockdown, ventures are utilizing cloud capacities to check, keep up, and screen their server and capacity establishments in server farms. Organizations are utilizing the cloud successfully to make flexible and calamity-avoidance frameworks at anyplace over the globe to take into account a remote workforce and secure information and business application respectability, too. IT resources are profoundly receiving server farm administrations to improve security, maintain a strategic distance from others, organize vacation, and accomplish operational effectiveness. Driving players, for example, DataBank, alongside the assistance of administrative groups, have begun setting up a COVID-19 response intended to evaluate the progression of activities. In this manner, the inexorably portable workforce because of lockdowns, and developing requirements for debacle recuperation and security to keep away from high system time costs, have energized the interest in cloud benefits over the globe [58]. The way that current IoT applications can be repurposed to aid the COVID-19 danger is basic, as it implies that these demonstrated arrangements were accessible and fit to be utilized at the beginning of the infection flare-up. In such a manner, organizations from all areas of the IoT biological system ought to consider how their present arrangements can be strategically repurposed to help associations and governments in battling the pandemic.

Looking forward, the most significant job of IoT, as identified with COVID-19, is probably going to be one of counteraction and assisting with distinguishing the flare-ups before they arrive at a mass scale [62]. Ordered establishment of associated thermometers in air terminals could be an IoT application that, before long, gets typical. Another conceivable, however likely longer-term execution is a system of sensors that distinguish hints of COVID-19. Upon identification, an area could be "secured" to restrain spread and guarantee brief treatment to affected people. It's not very difficult to envision such frameworks being joined into future shrewd city organizations, which, as of now, incorporate applications planned for improving open healthcare, for example, weapon discharge identification and air quality sensors. Below, we describe various applicable areas associated with cloud and IoT.

2.6.1 APPLICATION OF CLOUD SERVICE

In light of the innovation, the cloud services model section of the market is anticipated to hold a bigger market size during the gauged time frame. With the ascent in the instances of COVID-19, cloud service models are confronting a generous hit. There are a great deal of verticals of cloud, for example, producing, shopper products, and retail, and so forth, where all the activities are required to be postponed. Yet, associations have changed their needs, for example, associations are using cloud robotization and expanding their online nearness by creating trade sites on cloud stages to diminish the effect of COVID-19 on profitability and operational effectiveness. Such use cases are advanced in this COVID-19 pandemic. Some new use cases have been created alongside application regions where the interest for the cloud service model has seen an extensive increment [15]. The development of the service models will be prudently affected by verticals, for example, transportation, coordination, and assembling. Since the reception of the cloud is less contrasted with different verticals, the disturbance due to COVID-19 will have a moderate effect. It will decrease the product arrangement's development to a lesser degree.

2.6.2 HEALTH CARE SEGMENT

The social insurance frameworks need an adaptable and safe cloud foundation to oversee and keep up data with high speed and adaptability. During the COVID-19 pandemic, there is a serious requirement for innovations, for example, distributed computing for the investigation of patients' information. As the quantity of electronic wellbeing records is expanding, social insurance suppliers are growing the utilization of adaptable and profoundly secure capacity clouds to take into account an enormous number of cases. Private specialists and medicinal service establishments are giving web-based counseling amid nation lockdowns. The requirement for portable walking administrations has expanded because of the infection flare-up [15]. These offices and administrations need cloud-based correspondence and joint effort stages to improve operational proficiency and representative profitability. Human services suppliers are creating cloud-based applications to increase clinical experiences on COVID-19 and gauge asset necessities, for example, ICU beds and ventilators. Along these lines, expanded information investigation and clinical understanding necessities, and high spending on cloud-based application improvement and ERP arrangements amid the COVID-19 pandemic are making income open doors for cloud specialist organizations.

2.6.3 TRACKING THE SPREAD

Another job of cloud big data is following of the COVID-19 spread, which is of central significance for human services associations and governments in effectively controlling the coronavirus pandemic [15]. Various recently developing arrangements utilizing huge information have been proposed to help the following of the COVID-19 spread. For example, the investigation in [63] recommended a major information-based technique for following the COVID-19 spread. A different direct model is assembled utilizing nearby populace and air travelers as evaluated factors that are valuable to measure the change of announced cases in urban communities. All the more explicitly, the creators utilized a Spearman relationship examination for the everyday client traffic from the contaminated city and the all-out client traffic in this period, with the quantity of 49 affirmed cases. The investigative outcomes show a high relationship between the positive disease cases and the populace size. The creators in [64] thought about utilizing both enormous information for spatial investigation strategies and Geographic Information Systems (GIS) innovation, which would encourage information obtaining and the combination of heterogeneous information from wellbeing information assets, for example, governments, patients, clinical labs, and the general population.

2.6.4 DIAGNOSIS

Notwithstanding the forecast and spread using cloud infrastructure, the cloud can bolster COVID-19 determination and treatment forms. Truth be told, the capability of the cloud resource for diagnosing irresistible sicknesses like COVID-19 has been demonstrated through late victories, from early findings [65], the expectation of treatment results, and building steady devices for a medical procedure. As to COVID-19 conclusion and treatment, cloud information has given different arrangements, as detailed in the writing. An investigation in [66] presented a vigorous, delicate, explicit, and profoundly quantitative arrangement dependent on multiplex polymerase chain responses that can analyze COVID-19. The model comprises of contained 172 sets of explicit groundworks related to the genome of SARS-CoV-2 that can be gathered from the Chinese National Center for Biological data. The proposed Multiplex PCR plot has been demonstrated to be a proficient and easy strategy to analyze Plasmodium falciparum contaminations, with a high inclusion median of 99% and a particularity of 99.8%. Another exploration, in [67], executed a molecular indicative technique for genomic investigations of SARS-CoV-2 strains, with attention on Australian returned voyagers with COVID-19 utilizing genome information. This investigation may give significant bits of knowledge into viral decent variety and backing COVID-19 conclusion in regions with lacking genomic information.

TABLE 2.11
Security Actions

Actions	Requirement for Satisfied Security	Delivering Method
Identification and scanning	• Authentication and confidentiality. • Availability. • Non-repudiation.	• Testing penetration manually. • Verification manually. • Foot-printing. • Scanning Vulnerability.
Authentication review and authorization	• Authentication and confidentiality. • Privacy. • Trust. • Availability.	• Authorization policies review. • Error handling and management exception review. • Cluster authentication and management review. • Users and session review. • Privilege issues and configuration identify.
Deployment control and configuration of clusters	• Predication and intrusion detection. • Time-criticality. • Authentication and confidentiality. • Availability.	• Data flow and control understand. • Patch management process and configuration review of cluster. • Big-Data implementation of identify architectural issues. • Logging and backup processes and monitoring review.
Planning big data security	• Predication and intrusion detection. • Time-criticality. • Authentication and confidentiality.	• Uncovering operational risks of Big-Data. • Sharing expertise concerning privacy and data risk.

2.7   SECURITY OF THE ALLOCATION OF RESOURCES

This segment is principally concentrated on the security of these resources in the cloud. Technical discipline and processes are used by IT organizations on security based on their cloud infrastructure. IT organizations outsource management in various perspectives like innovation stack, organizing model, servers, stockpiling, virtualization, working frameworks, middleware, runtime, information, and applications through a cloud specialist co-op. Cyber-attacks, data theft, and other forms of attack are security threats IT organizations focus on, keeping security in the cloud. Table 2.11 shows the security actions associated with security in the resources.

2.7.1   Security Aspect

Any secured resource allocation system has several security aspects that can ensure the efficient and accurate allocation of resources. This area is principally concentrated on angles and security prerequisites for allocation. Below, we make mention of the security aspect in resource allocation.

2.7.1.1 Confidentiality and Authentication

Ensuring data transmission between resources and users, a technique-based encryption is commonly collaborated to ensure a reliable storage of data. A requirement that is also essential is authentication; it is also important for resources to authenticate users for service/data access in the case of heterogeneous systems. Thus, intelligently verifying resources requested for transparency and reliability are key components which are not currently sufficient for identification and authentication methods [58].

2.7.1.2 Privacy

Frequent attacks, like malware in mobile apps and smart devices, are a big risk to Big-data servers, like information capturing, which leads to the leakage of sensitive data in wireless communications [62]. This is a big threat to user's privacy in some resources. Repurposed data, published data, and leaked data are ways used in hacking the privacy of the user. Anonymous and encryption techniques are proposed in countering these attacks and are proved to be effective.

2.7.1.3 Time-Necessity

Versatility factor is a criterion in considering a resource network with the expectation of strict constraints. Especially considering a time-sensitive data tolerating no mistake and which can make a shocking impact in an organisation, if not met conveniently. Time necessity is a huge criteria in organization to meet their needs on time.

2.7.1.4 Availability

Resources that can be gotten to at whatever point required essentially suggest availability. Even with the high threat of attack, resources should continue functioning. Thus, there should be a way hacks can be recognized to stop the attack. There should be a solid defense and adaptive techniques in encountering a security threat [15].

2.7.1.5 Trust

The trust factor is a primary component in a secure system resource. Human factors in independent devices/nodes in the cloud have a higher chance of expecting any misbehavior. There must be a form of trust between service providers and users, since users are adamant about their privacy. A third party inquires the authority which guarantees trust between users and service providers.

2.7.1.6 Predication and Intrusion Detection

Three methodologies for interruption detection are anomaly recognition, specification identification, and misuse discovery. Due to resource capabilities, development is to be done in these approaches. Thus, intrusions based on lightweight detection are to be reviewed and developed [63].

2.7.2 SECURITY ISSUES AND CHALLENGES

Cloud resource security has been a concern for IT organizations, as its deployment of applications in the cloud are increasing in numbers. New security issues and challenges are rising due to the introduction of the proliferation of cloud services which traditional network security techniques can't manage. Innovation and technology adoption is one of the driving, core challenges in cloud security today [64].

2.7.2.1   Data Protection in Cloud Environments

Physical access to the server control is being lost by the service provider to organizations that are choosing to host sensitive data. This creates a grey area in the security of these resources, because the organization lacks administrative control over who accesses the server. Accessing data illegally, modifying, or copying and distributing it to others can be done easily by an employee of the service provider [65]. Conduction of detailed background of employees is to be carried out by the service provider and transparent and strict access control to servers and IT infrastructure to prevent insider attacks.

2.7.2.2   Authentication of User and Management Access

Username and password must be a form of security in cloud resources. Login credentials can be stolen by a nefarious actor gaining unauthorized access or modifying data in cloud service. Malicious code can also be released into the system by an attacker. A secure credentialing and management access system is being implemented by service providers to ensure an effective security measure for users [66].

2.7.2.3   Lack of Visibility of Cloud Services

The absence of permeability of utilizations and administrations is one of the significant difficulties looked at by IT associations sent on the cloud. Effectively gathering or amassing information concerning the security status of users and frameworks conveyed in the cloud is essentially alluded to as the absence of permeability [67].

2.7.2.4   Absence of Control over Cloud Infrastructure

Concerning the IT legacy system managed and conveyed on-premises, unlimited authority is being maintained by IT organizations with administrative control over every entire technology stack concerning every piece of IT infrastructure. IT organizations will have to be reliant on cloud resource providers concerning administrative decisions including a high-security standard [68].

2.8   OPEN RESEARCH AND DISCUSSION

Research issues are open, including several challenges that are still undergoing study in literature; they inquire careful attention. One of them includes algorithms associated with resource allocation, scheduling, and security. In this era, transmitting a lot of information in a dependable and auspicious way is a foundation to be accomplished. Therefore, the impact of efficient allocation should be accurately analyzed. This facilitates an advantage in achieving maximum transmission rates, scheduling, security, and capacity of the channel. Therefore, researches need to be carried out in developing a novel technique in the relation between users and the resource to be used. Several paradigms have been integrated with relations to this technique on cloud volunteered computing, with these paradigms being integrated on the cloud; this will always be a significant open problem for research. Attackers can exploit a lack of efficient security measures to steal data by posing as a user. Thus, an efficient scheme of authentication, including data integrity, is guaranteed in the cloud for keeping personal information secured.

Modern cloud resources increase the techniques and programmability of implementing these resources to be more efficient. However, for the optimization of resources, several developed scheduling strategies have been used. Indeed, to optimize QoS, resources accessibility and handling have to be tracked directly, which bangs on energy utilizations. However, the administration of resources and energy saving is said to be the main challenge goal for efficient resource use.

Resource allocation is the way toward assigning assets accessible to customers as per their needs. It is also the assigning of resources available to cloud applications that need it over the internet. The significant expectation of the cloud resource suppliers and customers is to allocate the cloud assets productively. In cloud volunteered computing, the main goal in resource allocation is assigning resources to users in need over the internet. Another important criterion is that it can starve certain services if management is not done precisely. The problem is solved by the service provider by managing each resource; this is called resource provisioning.

The major significance of scheduling is on how efficiently the process is being managed and increasing performance for servers and resources. This is also referred to as the efficiency of scheduling mechanism. As we discussed earlier, each scheduling mechanism has their various problem, but maximizing efficiency is the main goal. We can say the major difference will depend on how efficiently each mechanism executes its objective. There is a requirement for an arrangement for planning which will be good for specialist co-ops, just as clients. As a piece of future research, there should be an implementation of scheduling policy based on cost.

A high volume of data being generated will fuel ML algorithms to diagnose, prognose, and predict the allocation of resources and find users in need. Even though great results have been achieved, there are still demanding issues that need to be addressed for adequately leveraging a full autonomous resource allocation scheme, such as adversarial attacks and standards in evaluating and training ML algorithms, specifically in the cloud. The open research issues are to be considered in solving these issues and ensure the reliable deployment of ML models in the cloud.

2.9 CONCLUSION

Nowadays, cloud volunteered computing resources have been getting a great deal of consideration due to the new generation technology. A lot of the hardware and software resources are being provided to users based on their demands. In this survey paper, we gave a review of resource allocation and also considered its architectures, types, scheduling, intelligence issues, and security in the field. We also discussed challenges associated with some resources' communication and entity roles in the cloud volunteered computing. We also discussed the efficiency of these resources. We shed some light on some discussion and an insight into some open issues in research such as some critical scheduling algorithms and allocation algorithms. In future works, we will improve and see how the resources can be implemented to be more efficient with new resource allocation algorithms. This survey is believed to overpower faced difficulties.

REFERENCES

1. David Anderson, P. (2010). Volunteer computing: The ultimate cloud. *Crossroads*, 16(3), 7–10. [Online] Available: https://doi.org/10.1145/1734160.1734164.
2. Mell, P., and T. Grance. (2011). The NIST definition of cloud computing. *National Institute of Standards and Technology Special Publication*, NIST (pp. 800–145).
3. Lin, W., B. Peng, C. Liang, and B. Liu. (2013). Novel resource allocation model & algorithm for cloud computing. In Fourth International Conference on Emerging Intelligent Data and Web Technologies (EIDWT). IEEE.
4. Gokilavani, M., S. Selvi, and C. Udhaya kumar. (2013). A survey on resource allocation and task scheduling algorithms in cloud environment. *International Journal of Engineering and Innovative Technology (IJEIT)*, 3(4), pp: 173-179.
5. Pradeep, R., and R. Kavinya. (2012). Resource scheduling in cloud using bee algorithm for heterogeneous environment. *IOSR Journal of Computer Engineering (IOSRJCE)*, 2(4), 15–16.
6. Ventresca, M., and B. M. Ombuki. (2004). Ant colony optimization for job scheduling problem. *Journal of Mathematical Model and Algorithms*, 3(3), 285–308.
7. Rouse, M. (2016). Cloud storage. [Online]. Available: https://www.techtarget.com/contributor/Margaret-Rouse.
8. Mitchell, B. (2019). Computer network storage explained. [Online], Available: https://www.lifewire.com/what-is-computer-networking-816249.
9. Singh, H. (2012). Cloud computing: An internet based computing. *International Journal of Computers & Technology*,2(3), 116–121..
10. V. Suruchee Nandgaonkar, and A. B. Raut. A comprehensive study on cloud computing. *International Journal of Computer Science and Mobile Computing (IJCSMC)*,3(4),. 733–738.
11. Sriram, l., and A. Khajeh Hossani. (2010). *Research Agenda in Cloud Computing Technologies*. Dept. of Computer Science, University of Bristol.
12. Hu, F., and M. Qin. A review on cloud computing: Design challenges in architecture and security. *Journal of Computing and Information Technology (JCIT)*, 1, 25–55.
13. Chawla, Y., and M. Bhonsle. (2012). A study on scheduling methods in cloud computing. *International Journal of Emerging Trends & Technology in Computer Science (IJETTCS)*, 1(3), 12–17.
14. Tripathy, L., and R. R. Patra. (2014). Scheduling in cloud computing. *International Journal on Cloud Computing: Services and Architecture (IJCCSA)*, 4(5), ISSN 2277-8616.
15. MarketsandMarkets. (2020). Is big data effective in response to coronavirus outbreak? [Online]. Available: https://www.analyticsinsight.net/big-data-effective-response-coronavirus-outbreak/.
16. Al-Turjman, Fadi, Mohammed Hasan, and Hussain Al-Rizzo. (2018). Task scheduling in cloud-based survivability applications using swarm optimization in IoT. *Transactions on Emerging Telecommunications Technologies*, e3539. 10.1002/ett.3539.
17. Xue, S. (2014). An improved algorithm based on NSGA-II for cloud PDTs scheduling. *Journal of Software*, 6, 443–450.

18. Gomathi, B., and K. Karthikeyan. (2013). Task scheduling algorithm based on hybrid particle swarm optimization in cloud computing environment. *Journal of Theoretical and Applied Information Technology*, 89, 33–38.

19. Kaur, N., T. S. Aulakh, and R. S. Cheema. (2011). Comparison of workflow scheduling algorithms in cloud computing. *International Journal of Advanced Computer Science and Applications (IJACSA)*, 2(10), 146–148.

20. Wang, W., and G. Zeng. (2011). Trusted dynamic scheduling for large-scale parallel distributed systems. In International Conference on Parallel Processing Workshops, ICPPW 2011, Taipei, Taiwan. IEEE.

21. Salimi, R., H. Motameni, and H. Omranpour. Task scheduling using NSGA II with fuzzy adaptive operators for computational grids. *Journal of Parallel and Distributed Computing*, 74, 2333–2350.

22. Cheng, B.. (2012). Hierarchical cloud service workflow scheduling optimization schema using heuristic generic algorithm. *Telecommunications*, 15, 92–95.

23. Pandey, S., L. Wu, S. Guru, and R. Buyya. (2010). A particle swarm optimization based heuristic for scheduling workflow applications in cloud computing environments. In 24th IEEE International Conference on Advanced Information Networking and Applications (pp. 400–407). IEEE.

24. Wu, L. (2012). *A Revised Discrete Particle Swarm Optimization for Cloud Workflow Scheduling* (pp. 1–5). Faculty of Information and Communication Technologies Swinburne University of Technology.

25. Zhao, S., X. Lu, and X. Li. (2015). Quality of service-based particle swarm optimization in cloud computing. *Computer Engineering and Networks*, 8, 235–242.

26. Izakian, H., B. Ladani, A. Abraham, and V. Snasel. (2014). A discrete particle swarm optimization approach for grid job scheduling. *International Journal of Innovative Computing Information and Control*, 16, 4219–4252.

27. Banerjee, S., I. Mukherjee, and P. Mahanti. (2009). Cloud computing initiative using modified ant colony framework. *World Academy of Science, Engineering and Technology*, 12, 200–203.

28. Zaharia, M., D. Borthakur, J. Sen Sarma, K. Elmeleegy, S. Shenker, and I. Stoica. (2010). Delay scheduling: A simple technique for achieving locality and fairness in cluster scheduling. In Proceedings of the 5th European Conference on Computer systems (EuroSys). *Association for Computing Machinery, New York, NY, USA, 265–278.* DOI: 10.1145/1755913.1755940.

29. Ludwig, S., and A. Moallem. (2013). Swarm intelligence approaches for grid load balancing. *Journal of Grid Computing*, 8, 279–301.

30. Al-Turjman, F., and I. Baali. (2019). Machine learning for wearable IoT-based applications: A survey. *Article in Transactions on Emerging Telecommunications Technologies*, e3635. DOI: 10.1002/ett.3635.

31. Mousavi, S. M., and G. Fazekas. (2016). A novel algorithm for load balancing using HBA and ACO in cloud computing environment. *International Journal of Computer Science and Information Security*, 16, 48–52.

32. Dhinesh Babu, L. D., and P. V. Krishna. (2013). Honey bee behavior inspired load balancing of tasks in cloud computing environments. *Applied Soft Computing*, 13, 2292–2303.

33. Abdullah, M., and M. Othman. (2014). Simulated annealing approach to cost based multi-quality of service job scheduling in cloud computing environment. *American Journal of Applied Sciences*, 18, 872–877.

34. Henzinger, T. A., A. V. Singh, V. Singh, T. Wies, D. Zufferey. (2011). Static scheduling in clouds. *Memory*, 200, i1, 329–342.

35. Lee, Z., Y. Wang, and W. Zhou. (2011). A dynamic priority scheduling algorithm on service request scheduling in cloud computing. In Proceedings of 2011 International Conference on Electronic and Mechanical Engineering and Information Technology, EMEIT, Harbin, Heilongjiang, China. IEEE.
36. Zhao, L., Y. Ren, Y. Xiang, and K. Sakurai. (2011). Fault-tolerant scheduling with dynamic number of replicas in heterogeneous systems. In Proceedings of the 12th IEEE International Conference on High Performance Computing and Communications (pp. 434–441). IEEE.
37. Li, J., M. Qiu, J. Niu, W. Gao, Z. Zong, and X. Qin. (2010). Feedback dynamic algorithms for preemptable job scheduling in cloud systems. In EEE/WIC/ACM International Conference on Web Intelligence and Intelligent Agent Technology. IEEE.
38. Cao, Q., Z.-B. Wei, and W.-M. Gong. (2009). An optimized algorithm for task scheduling based on activity based costing in cloud computing. In 2010 IEEE/WIC/ACM International Conference on Web Intelligence and Intelligent Agent Technology. IEEE.
39. Zinnen, A., and T. Engel. (2011). Deadline constrained scheduling in hybrid clouds with Gaussian processes. In International Conference on High Performance Computing and Simulation (HPCS). IEEE.
40. Suresh, A., and P. Vijayakarthick. (2011). Improving scheduling of backfill algorithms using balanced spiral method for cloud meta scheduler. In IEEE-International Conference on Recent Trends in Information Technology, ICRTIT. IEEE.
41. Zhao, L., Y. Ren, and K. Sakurai. (2011). A resource minimizing scheduling algorithm with ensuring the deadline and reliability in heterogeneous systems. In Proceedings: 25th IEEE International Conference on Advanced Information Networking and Applications, AINA. IEEE.
42. Yang, B., X. Xu, F. Tan, D. and H. Park. (2012). A utility-based job scheduling algorithm for Cloud computing considering reliability factor. In International Conference on Cloud and Service Computing. IEEE.
43. Jin, J., J. Luo, A. Song, F. Dong, and R. Xiong. (2011). Bar: An efficient data locality driven task scheduling algorithm for cloud computing. In 11th IEEE/ACM International Symposium on Cluster, Cloud and Grid Computing. IEEE.
44. Bo, Z., G. Ji, and A. Jieqing. (2011). Cloud loading balance algorithm. In The 2nd International Conference on Information Science and Engineering. IEEE.
45. Frincu, M.E., and C. Craciun. (2012). Multi-objective meta heuristics for scheduling applications with high availability requirements and cost constraints in multi cloud environments. In Proceedings of the IEEE 18th International Conference on Utility and Cloud Computing (pp. 267–274). IEEE.
46. Tang, L., C. Zhu, W. Zhang, and Z. Liu. (2011). Robust COA planning with varying durations. In IEEE International Conference on Cloud Computing and Intelligence Systems. IEEE.
47. Zhu, K., H. Song, L. Liu, J. Gao, and G. Cheng. (2012). Hybrid genetic algorithm for cloud computing applications. In 2011 IEEE Asia-Pacific Services Computing Conference. IEEE.
48. Zhao, C., S. Zhang, Q. Liu, J. Xie, and J. Hu. (2009). Independent tasks scheduling based on genetic algorithm in cloud computing. In 5th International Conference on Wireless Communications, Networking and Mobile Computing (pp. 5548–5551). IEEE.
49. Liu, S., G. Quan, and S. Ren. (2010). On-line scheduling of real-time services for cloud computing. In 6th World Congress on Services. IEEE.
50. Liu, S., G. Quan, and S. Ren. (2011). On-line preemptive scheduling of real-time services with profit and penalty. IEEE International Conference on Service-Oriented Computing and Applications (SOCA) (287–292). IEEE.

51. Gu, Y., and Y. Ge. (2010). A real-time workload driven approach for the cloud. In Second International Conference on Modeling, Simulation and Visualization Methods. IEEE.
52. Zhu, X., J. Zhu, M. Ma, and D. Qiu. (2010). SAQA: A self-adaptive QoS-aware scheduling algorithm for real-time tasks on heterogeneous clusters. In 10th IEEE/ACM International Conference on Cluster, Cloud and Grid Computing. IEEE.
53. Yu, Z., and W. Shi. (2008). A planner-guided scheduling strategy for multiple workflow applications. In International Conference on Parallel Processing Workshops (pp. 1–8). IEEE.
54. Yu, J., and R. Buyya. (2007). Workflow scheduling algorithms for grid computing. Technical Report, GRIDS-TR-2007-10. Grid Computing and Distributed Systems Laboratory, The University of Melbourne, Australia.
55. Bala, A., and I. Chana. (2011). A survey of various workflow scheduling algorithms in cloud environment. In 2nd National Conference on Information and Communication Technology (NCICT). *IJCA Journal*, 4, 26–30.
56. Liu, K. (2009). *Scheduling Algorithms for Instance Intensive Cloud Workflows.* Swinburne University of Technology.
57. Narman, H. S., M. S. Hossain, and M. Atiquzzaman. (2014). h-DDSS: Heterogeneous dynamic dedicated servers scheduling in cloud computing. In IEEE International Conference on Communications (ICC). IEEE.
58. MarketsandMarkets. (2020). COVID-19 impact on cloud computing market. [Online] Available: https://www.prnewswire.com/news-releases/covid-19-impact-on-cloud-computing-market--exclusive-report-by-marketsandmarkets-301047436.html.
59. Merkle, D., and M. Middendorf. (2003). Ant colony optimization with global pheromone evaluation for scheduling a single machine. *Applied Intelligence*, 18(1), 105–111.
60. Guo, L., S. Zhao, S. Shen, and C. Jiang. (2012). Task scheduling optimization in cloud computing based on heuristic algorithm. In *IEEE Journal of Networks*, 7(3), p. 547.
61. Liu, X., C. Wang, B. B. Zhou, J. Chen, T. Yang, and A. Y. Zomaya. (2013). Priority-based consolidation of parallel workloads in the cloud. *IEEE Transactions on Parallel and Distributed Systems*, 24(9), 1874–1883.
62. MarketsandMarkets. (2020). COVID-19 impact on cloud computing market service model. [Online] Available: https://www.marketsandmarkets.com/Market-Reports/covid-19-impact-on-cloud-computing-market-86614844.html.
63. Zhao, X., X. Liu, and X. Li. (2020). Tracking the spread of novel coronavirus (2019-ncov) based on big data. *medRxiv*. DOI: 10.1101/2020.02.07.20021196.
64. Zhou, C., F. Su, T. Pei, A. Zhang, Y. Du, B. Luo, Z. Cao, J. Wang, W. Yuan, and Y. Zhu. (2020). COVID-19: Challenges to GIS with big data. *Geography and Sustainability*, 1(1), 77–87.
65. Garattini, C., J. Raffle, D. N. Aisyah, F. Sartain, and Z. Kozlakidis. (2019). Big data analytics, infectious diseases and associated ethical impacts. *Philosophy & Technology*, 32(1), 69–85.
66. Li, C., D. N. Debruyne, J. Spencer, V. Kapoor, L. Y. Liu, B. Zhou, L. Lee, R. Feigelman, G. Burdon, and J. Liu. (2020). High sensitivity detection of coronavirus SARS-CoV-2 using multiplex PCR and a multiplex-PCR-based metagenomic method. *bioRxiv*. DOI: 10.1101/2020.03.12.988246.
67. Eden, J.-S., R. Rockett, I. Carter, H. Rahman, J. de Ligt, J. Hadfield, M. Storey, X. Ren, R. Tulloch, and K. Basile. An emergent clade of SARS-CoV-2 linked to returned travellers from Iran. *bioRxiv*. DOI: 10.1101/2020.03.15.992818.
68. Kreuter, D. (2004). Where server virtualization was born. *International Journal of Advance Research in Computer Science and Management Studies*, 2(4), 15–23.

3 Analyzing Radiographs for COVID-19 Using Artificial Intelligence

Manpreet Sirswal, Ekansh Chauhan,
Deepak Gupta, Ashish Khanna,
and Fadi Al-Turjman

CONTENTS

3.1   INTRODUCTION

COVID-19, or the novel coronavirus, has created immense havoc across the world. The coronavirus was first introduced in the 1960s. It was known to cause infection in the respiratory tracts of children. Then it started surfacing in 2003, causing a significant number of deaths; this virus was named SARS-CoV-1. It brought zoonotic viruses, i.e. the viruses that spread from animals to humans, into the limelight. Human isolation was enough to eradicate them and to contain their spread. Then, a virus called MERS came into existence in 2012–2013. It was also stopped from spreading just by following human isolation guidelines. Now, in December 2019, strange pneumonia cases were reported which were later identified as COVID-19 which is caused by SARS-CoV-2, also a zoonotic virus [1]. One thing that is common in all of these zoonotic viruses is that they all trigger respiratory diseases. SARS-CoV-2 is a single strand RNA virus which is very easily transmissible from humans to humans. It was declared a pandemic in March 2020 by the WHO. A lot of research is being conducted to develop drugs and a vaccine against coronavirus. No cure is available currently. Several health and social distancing guidelines are issued by the governments of countries and the WHO to curb its spread. Early diagnosis of the patients is the only way of suppressing the virus, as a lot of infected people are asymptomatic, i.e. they don't show any symptoms of having coronavirus, which is very difficult for countries with poor healthcare systems. Conventional laboratory testing is very time consuming and expensive, and it also puts the healthcare workers at a risk of getting infected [2]. There is an urgent need for quick and reliable methods of testing and classifying patients who need immediate treatment. Machine learning (ML) and deep learning have solved many complex problems in the past, and at this time of pandemic, they can contribute by training their models on radiograph images to detect and diagnose the disease rapidly, hence making this critical task easier [3]. They can predict if the patient is in risk zone or safe zone quite accurately.

The main objective of this chapter is to form a parallel system of diagnosing by designing a neural network using machine learning and deep learning; therefore, the main focus is on using Artificial Intelligence (AI) technology to fight against COVID-19. Public data of X-rays and CT scans was taken from various sources such as GitHub, Radiopaedia, and Kaggle for the analysis. Images of X-rays are also used with CT scans for parallel analysis, because in countries with major rural populations, X-ray labs are relatively easier and cheaper to set up in comparison to CT scan labs, and the cost of X-ray scanning is less as compared to CT scanning, which makes it easily accessible to a lot of rural or poor people. So, collected data of X-ray images of healthy and COVID-19–infected patients was put into three models: VGG-16, VGG-19, and custom model [4]. The analysis of this data was done with a machine learning tool called CNN. CNN models were used to classify the COVID-19 infected chest X-rays and normal chest X-rays. Activation maps were used to outline the infected area of the CT and X-ray scans. For CT scans, machine learning and deep learning was used to extract the graphical features of the several COVID-19 positive patients, thus training the model for coronavirus identification. Then, the convolutional neural network was used on the dataset of CT scan images of infected patients. All these ciphering techniques are a part of Artificial Intelligence systems. Any new piece of information is of immense value to both the humans and the Artificial Intelligence systems.

This chapter is distributed in different sections. In Section 3.2, the view and work of other researchers who have done similar work for contribution to the analysis of COVID-19 is discussed, and the dataset used and data augmentation are discussed in Section 3.3 and Section 3.4, respectively. In Section 3.5, the different methodologies implemented on the datasets for the classification of normal and COVID-19–infected patients are deliberated. Further, the results of all the models are compared and evaluated in Section 3.6. Finally, all of the work proposed in this chapter is concluded in the Section 3.7.

3.2 RELATED WORK

The first three cases of COVID-19 patients in France were considered in Ref. [5] by the authors. Two of them were diagnosed in Paris and one was diagnosed in Bordeaux. All of them had been living in Wuhan, China before coming to France. In Ref. [6], hybrid systems based on Artificial Intelligence were proposed by the authors. These hybrid systems used machine learning and deep learning algorithms like convoluted neural network (CNN), which was implemented to detect COVID-19 by distinguishing normal and COVID-19–infected chest X-rays.

A MERS- (Middle East respiratory syndrome) infected patient was analyzed in Ref. [7]. MERS is very closely related to the coronavirus family. The patient was 30 years old and had symptoms like diarrhea and abdominal pain. Authors gave an analysis of treatment of infected persons with chest X-ray. Further, they applied this model on a collected dataset of chest X-ray and CT images and received improved results. In Ref. [8], chest CT scans of 21 patients suffering from COVID-19 in Wuhan were analyzed. The main focus of the paper was to demonstrate the effect of the coronavirus on lungs. Finally, in Ref. [9], 50 COVID-19 positive patients were distributed into two categories of good and poor recovery. Identification of risk factor of weak recovery and lung infection was done. At the end, it was concluded that 58% patients have very poor chances of recovery.

3.3 DATASET

The data was assembled from 3 different sources to form a dataset of 283 X-ray images and 309 CT scan images. The number of images collected from their respective sources are portrayed in Table 3.1. The reasons of using these sources for the collection of dataset are that these sources contain images of very diverse people from different countries, which is very important for helping radiologists to diagnose COVID-19 across the globe, and the images from all of these sources are available publicly, to the general public and other researchers. The X-ray images for COVID-19 positive patients were taken from the GitHub repository [10], however, this repository contains very vast data, out of which a very small amount of data is of our use; therefore, we have selected the "finding" column=COVID-19, "view" = PA, and "modality" = X-ray. Then, using the shutil library of Python they were all combined to form an efficient dataset. This gave us 133 X-ray images of COVID-19-positive patients. For CT scans of COVID-19 patients, the two GitHub

TABLE 3.1
Dataset Distribution

Mode ↓/Source →		GitHub	Kaggle	Radiopaedia
X-ray	COVID-19	133	----	----
	Normal	----	150	----
CT- Scan	COVID-19	25 + 131	----	----
	Normal	----	----	153

repositories were used, but with the "finding" column = COVID-19, "view" = axial, and "modality" = CT, which resulted in 25 CT scans, which were taken from Societa Italiana di Radiologia Medica e Interventistica (SIRM) (Italian Society of Medical Radiology and Interventional), and 131 images of COVID-19 patients were taken from another GitHub repository [11]. Further, 150 X-ray images and 153 CT scan images of healthy people were taken from Kaggle and Radiopaedia, respectively [12, 13]. All images were resized to 224 by 224 by 3 RGB images, which is width-by-height-by-channel number. We cropped the lung and chest area, such that it does not contain any writing, as much as possible. Figure 3.1 shows the example of data that is applied to our models. Both the datasets are being updated regularly. The patient

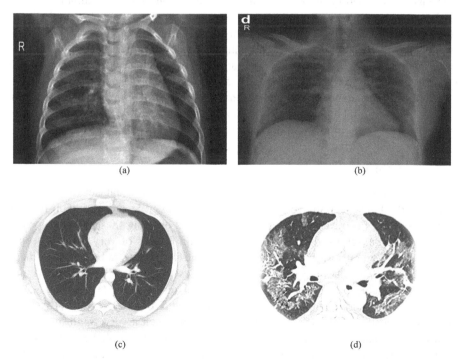

(a)   (b)

(c)   (d)

FIGURE 3.1 Dataset samples a) normal X-ray b) COVID-19 X-ray c) normal CT scan d) COVID-19 CT scan.

ages range from 12 to 84 years old, with genders mixed. The datasets are divided into two categories in the training phase, i.e. training set and test set.

Accuracy of the result is defined as $\dfrac{TP+TN}{\text{Total images tested}}$

Sensitivity is defined as $\dfrac{TP}{TP+FN}$.

And specificity is defined as $\dfrac{TN}{TN+FP}$

Where,
TP = true positive
TN = true negative
FP = false positive
FN = False negative

Accuracy, sensitivity and specificity are used as performance measures in this study.

3.4   DATA AUGMENTATION

Data collected from different sources needs to be cleaned before it is given as an input. Machine learning requires a large amount of datasets to produce reliable results, and it is possible that every problem does not have enough data, and in fact, it can be very expensive and time consuming to collect medical data. To solve these kinds of issues, data augmentation is used. According to [CNN], "Data Augmentation technique is a method that can artificially magnify the size of training dataset by formatting or resizing the image in a dataset." The augmentation techniques include rotation, zooming, and sharing of images. It helps to overcome the problem of overfitting [14, 15]. Data augmentation technique is used to find the retrospective experiments by testing the lung CT scan and X-ray images of the patient to detect the coronavirus disease. Hence, the prepared dataset, by implementing data augmentation, is used to train the models. It also helps in establishing models and enhances outcomes by statistical learning. Data augmentation technique has been used in machine learning for a very long time, and it has been acknowledged as a crucial investigating element of several models. This technique has made massive progress in classifying and segmenting images. Thus, data augmentation enhances the accuracy of classification and prediction models. It helps in producing effective results in much less computational time.

3.5   MODELS

3.5.1   VGG-16

VGG-16 is a convolutional neural network which is specifically trained for more than a million types of images, with respect to the dataset "ImageNet" [16]. This neural network is 16 layers deep and was first introduced by Simonyan and Zisserman in their study, "Very Deep Convolutional Networks for Large Scale Image Recognition," [17] and was developed by a visual geometry group from Oxford. This model has an accuracy of 92.7% in "ImageNet." We decided to choose this model so that we could avoid choosing other complex models, since our data is small. Figure 3.2 shows the architecture of the VGG-16 model. The size of the VGG-16 network, in terms of fully connected nodes, is 533 MB.

3.5.2   VGG-19

VGG-19 is also a convolutional neural network that is specifically trained for more than a million types of images with respect to the dataset "ImageNet." This neural network is 19 layers deep, as compared to the 16 layers of VGG -16, and was also first introduced by Simonyan and Zisserman in their study, "Very Deep Convolutional Networks for Large Scale Image Recognition," and was developed by the visual geometry group from Oxford. We decided to choose this model so that we could avoid choosing other complex models, since our data is small. Figure 3.3 shows the architecture of the VGG-19 model. The size of the VGG-19 network, in terms of fully connected nodes, is 574 MB.

3.5.3   CUSTOM MODEL

We have proposed a model in addition to the above models for the classification of X-ray images. This model gives almost identical performance to the above-mentioned models. This permits us to train the model quicker and decreases the inference time. Figure 3.4 depicts the architecture of our custom model.

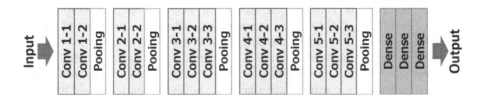

FIGURE 3.2   VGG-16 architecture.

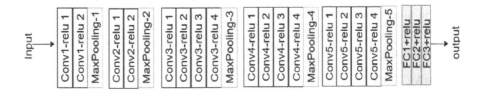

FIGURE 3.3   VGG-19 architecture.

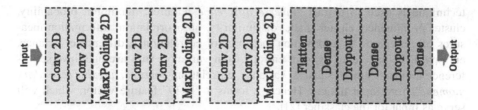

FIGURE 3.4 Custom model architecture.

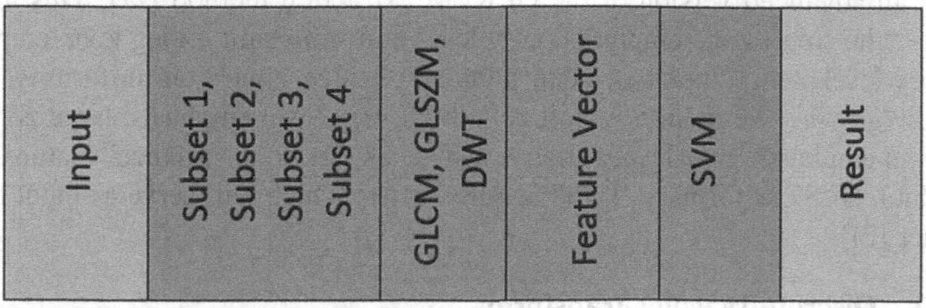

FIGURE 3.5 Classification process.

3.5.4 SVM

This model works in two stages; firstly, features are extracted to form feature vectors, using GLCM, GLSZM, and DWT. The feature vectors obtained are used for classification of coronavirus. For classification, SVM classifier is used, because it is considered a "strong binary" classifier [18]. SVM gives very high accuracy for the classification process in a lot of applications. SVM works on two main plans; the first one is to classify the data in high dimensional space using linear classifiers, and the second is to classify the data with high margin hyperplane. The value of cost parameter (C) is 1, by default, for all the classification processes in SVM. In this SVM model, we have converted all the CT scan images into subsets of 16×16, 32×32, 48×48, and 64×64 patches. Figure 3.5 depicts the classification of this model. Then, various techniques were used to extract features from these patches. The techniques are:

- Grey Level Co-Occurrence Matrix (GLCM).
- Grey Level Size Zone Matrix (GLSZM).
- Discrete Wavelet Transform (DWT).

3.5.4.1 Grey Level Co-Occurrence Matrix

This method is used to acquire the second-degree statistical features on images [19]. It derives the correlation between the different angles in the pixels of the image. A co-occurrence matrix is computed from an image scan and is depicted as $P = [p(i, j \mid d, \theta)]$; this means that i'th pixel frequency features are being evaluated with j'th pixel frequency features. θ represents the direction and d is the length [20]. This technique is used to extract *"inverse difference* features, maximum probability, cluster prominence, cluster shade, dissimilarity, autocorrelation, information measures of correlation 2, information measures of correlation 1, difference variance, entropy, difference entropy, sum entropy, sum variance, sum average, inverse difference moment, sum of squares: variance, correlation, contrast, *angular secondary moment"* from input images. Hence, it forms a "1×19" feature vector, which will serve as input for the classifier [21].

3.5.4.2   Grey Level Size Zone Matrix

This is an advanced version of the GLRLM extraction method [22]. This method extracts "the small zone emphasis, grey-level non-uniformity, long zone emphasis, low grey-level zone emphasis, zone percentage, size zone non-uniformity, small zone low grey-level emphasis, small zone high grey-level emphasis, large zone low grey-level emphasis, grey-level variance as well as size zone variance" features from input data. GLSZM forms a "1*13" feature vector, which will serve as input for the classifier [21].

3.5.4.3   Discrete Wavelet Transform

DWT divides the images into sub bands of frequency using h low pass filter and g high pass filter. "Diagonal details, vertical details, horizontal details, approximation co-efficient" represent the high frequency, vertical frequency, horizontal high frequency and lowest frequencies in both the directions respectively. LL coefficients produce the feature set and are hence converted into a "1×4" feature vector [23].

3.5.5   Modified CNN

To classify COVID-19-positive CT scans and normal CT scans, a very lucid CNN model is constructed. It is made up of one convolution layer, which has 16 filters in it, along with batch normalization, rectified linear unit (ReLU), fully connected layer, SoftMax, and a classification layer. The detailed image of the architecture of our modified CNN is shown in Figure 3.6.

3.5.5.1   Input Layer

This layer is in charge of reading all the input data. It includes a pre-processing step that crops and resizes the input CT scan images; because the images are taken

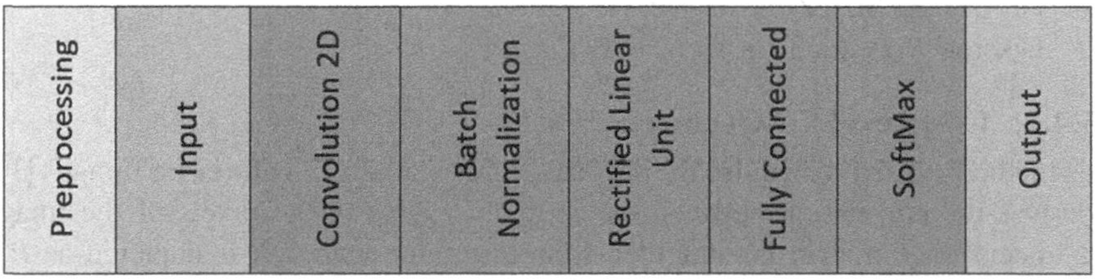

FIGURE 3.6   Modified CNN architecture.

from medical centers, there can be letters or symbols written on them, and since the images are taken from different sources, they can be of different sizes. The main aim of this pre-processing step is to crop the lung and chest area and to resize the images so that no text or symbol is written on the image.

3.5.5.2 Convolution Layer

This is the most important layer of our model, because it identifies the relationship between the pixels of the input image. The main aim of this layer is to extract features from the input image, which is done by learning the extracted features using various filters. This layer used 16 two-dimensional features which were made based on a 5×5 filter size. After extracting features and converting them into vectors, the filters also compute the dot product of all the features. CNN learns these features during the training phase, and all the convolved images and input images are of same size.

3.5.5.3 Batch Normalization Layer

This layer normalizes the extracted or convoluted feature values by using a very deep neural network training technique. This is mainly done to reduce the training stages, which is essential for stabilizing the training process.

3.5.5.4 Rectified Linear Unit Layer

The responsibility of the ReLU layer is to replace the negative pixel values by 0 in the convolved features. It is done in a CNN network for the features to have a non-linearity map.

3.5.5.5 Fully Connected layer

The main aim of this layer is to form defined classes of the extracted features from the input images. All the neurons of this layer are connected to activation functions of previous layer.

3.5.5.6 SoftMax Layer

This layer classifies the diagnosed cases into the two classes of "0" and "1." It calculates the possible values of activation function from previous layers.

3.5.5.7 Output

This is the last layer of the CNN network. It labels the images of CT scans with possible result values. For instance, a CT scan of a COVID-19-positive patient is labelled as "1," and a CT scan of a non-COVID-19 patient is labelled as "0."

3.6 RESULT AND ANALYSIS

3.6.1 VGG-16

VGG-16 is a CNN-based architecture that has 16 layers. It has "Convolutional layers, Activation layers, Max Pooling layers, and fully connected layers.". In this model, the X-ray dataset was trained on 80% data and tested on 20% data; shuffling of data

TABLE 3.2
VGG-16 Result

	Training Dataset			Testing Dataset		
Label	Precision	Recall	F1-Score	Precision	Recall	F1-Score
COVID-19	0.98	0.95	0.96	1.0	0.85	0.92
Normal	0.95	0.98	0.97	0.88	1.0	0.94
Accuracy			0.97			0.93

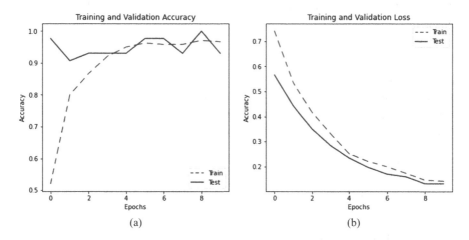

(a)   (b)

FIGURE 3.7   (a) Training and validation accuracy of VGG-16 (b) Training and validation loss of VGG-16 model.

was turned on. In the case of training, the result of sensitivity is 0.954, and specificity is 0.982, and in the case of testing, the result of sensitivity is 0.885, and specificity is 1.0, as shown in Table 3.2 and Figure 3.7.

3.6.2   VGG-19

VGG-19 is a variant of the VGG model that consists of 19 layers. In this model, "13 are convolutional layers where three are fully connected layer, 5 are Max Pool layers and one softmax layer." In this model, the X-ray dataset was trained on 80% data and tested on 20% data; shuffling of data was turned on. In training, the result of sensitivity is 1.0, and specificity is 0.983, and in the case of the training dataset, sensitivity is 1.0, and specificity is 1.0, as shown in Table 3.3 and Figure 3.8.

3.6.3   Custom Model

In this custom model, a collected dataset of healthy and COVID-19 X-ray image were trained and tested. In training, the result of sensitivity is 0.96, and specificity

TABLE 3.3
VGG-19 Result

Label	Training Dataset			Testing Dataset		
	Precision	Recall	F1-Score	Precision	Recall	F1-Score
COVID-19	0.98	1.0	0.99	1.0	1.0	1.0
Normal	1.0	0.98	0.99	1.0	1.0	1.0
Accuracy			0.99			1.0

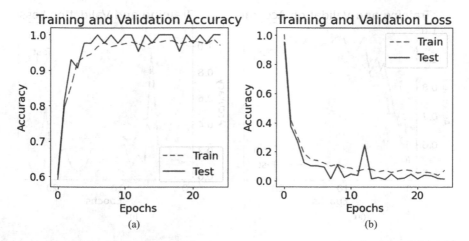

FIGURE 3.8 (a) Training and validation accuracy of the custom model (b) Training and validation loss of a VGG-19 model.

is 0.93. In the case of the training dataset, sensitivity is 1.0, and specificity is 1.0, as shown in Table 3.4 and Figure 3.9.

We can see that VGG-19 has the best performance among all the discussed models for the classification of X-rays.

3.6.4 SVM

Table 3.5 shows the best feature extraction method for each subset. All of the methods that we used, i.e. GLCM, GLSZM, DWT, had a classification accuracy of more than 90% during 10-fold cross validation. The best classification was attained by DWT during 10-fold cross validation. The strategy of the best method is depicted in Figure 3.10.

The CT image was converted into 48×48 sized patches. DWT extracts the features of the patches and forms a feature vector. Then, 10 different SVM structures classify the vector, which were formed during the training phase. The average classification performance is obtained by SVM.

TABLE 3.4

Custom Model Result

Label	Training dataset			Testing dataset		
	Precision	Recall	F1-score	Precision	Recall	F1-score
Covid-19	0.93	0.96	0.94	1.0	1.0	1.0
Normal	0.96	0.94	0.95	1.0	1.0	1.0
Accuracy			0.95			1.0

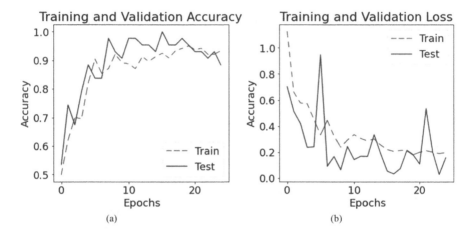

FIGURE 3.9 (a) Training and validation accuracy of the custom model (b) Training and validation loss of a custom model.

3.6.5 MODIFIED CNN

The modified CNN network achieved 90% sensitivity, 100% specificity, and 94.1% accuracy. This signifies that the modified, simpler CNN is performing very well in identifying the CT scans of COVID-19 patients and healthy patients.

All of our results show the efficiency of all the models that we've used for x-rays and CT scans in the classification of COVID-19-positive patients. This will immensely help the radiologists by reducing the load on doctors and healthcare systems.

3.7 ACTIVATION MAPS

This is a technique that is used to improve the results and accuracy of CNN-based networks, and makes them more transparent by visualizing the important regions for prediction during the classification process [24]. The equation responsible for this visualization is:

$$\alpha_k^c = \overbrace{\frac{1}{Z} \sum_i \sum_j}^{\text{global average pooling}} \underbrace{\frac{\partial y^c}{\partial A_{ij}^k}}_{\text{gradients via backprop}}$$

TABLE 3.5
Feature Extraction Result

Subset	Feature Extraction	Number of Features	Cross Validation	Sensitivity	Specificity	Accuracy	Precision	F-Score
1	GLCM	19	10-fold	98.52	99.23	98.91	99.1	98.81
2	DWT	256	10-fold	99.15	99.55	99.37	99.47	99.31
3	DWT	576	10-fold	99.23	100	99.64	100	99.6
4	DWT	1024	10-fold	93.39	100	97.28	100	96.46

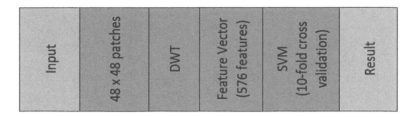

FIGURE 3.10 Optimum classification.

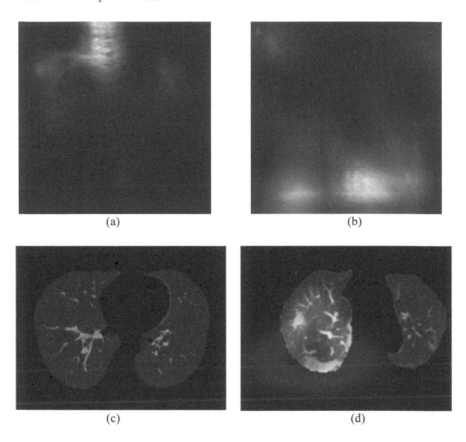

FIGURE 3.11 Activation maps a) normal X-ray b) COVID-19 X-ray c) normal CT scan d) COVID-19 CT scan.

The visualization achieved is of high resolution and is also class discriminative. The areas that are helping the model to classify the COVID-19 infected images more accurately are extracted using gradient-based activation maps [25]. Figure 3.11 shows the heat maps of the important or suspected areas for the identification of COVID-19 infection. It lays emphasis on the abnormal areas by highlighting them, while ignoring the normal regions as visualized in the figure.

3.8 CONCLUSION

The novel coronavirus was first identified in Wuhan, and within a span of 2–3 months, it spread all over the world. Economies of the biggest countries are crashing, thousands of people are dying, and lockdowns are imposed all over the world. AI, as usual, is playing its part in the fight against coronavirus. Early detection is the only way by which we can stop its spread. However, early detection is more difficult in this case, because a lot of the carriers of this virus are asymptomatic. Therefore, in this study, we took the data containing X-rays and CT scans of the lungs and chest of COVID-19-positive patients and healthy patients from different sources like GitHub and Kaggle. All of this data is publicly available to the research community. We then used different CNN models, like VGG-16, VGG-19, and a custom model, to classify the COVID-19 infected X-ray images and normal X-ray images. For the classification of CT-scans, an SVM classifier, along with feature extraction, and a modified, rather simple CNN model was used. Although very high accuracy of classification was achieved by most of our models, this does not mean that these models can be used as a solution for the detection of COVID-19, mostly due to the fact that the data used in these models was very limited. More classification and segmentation studies need to be done on COVID-19. The main aim of this study was to provide radiologists with potential models that can help in the early diagnosis of COVID-19 and might also help in accelerating the research in this direction.

REFERENCES

1. Rothan, H. A., and S. N. Byrareddy. (2020). The epidemiology and pathogenesis of coronavirus disease (COVID-19) outbreak. *Journal of Autoimmunity*, 109, 102433. doi: 10.1016/j.jaut.2020.102433.
2. Cohen, J. (2020). In bid to rapidly expand coronavirus testing, U.S. agency abruptly changes rules. *Science*, 80. doi: 10.1126/science.abb5231.
3. Alimadadi, A., S. Aryal, I. Manandhar, P. B. Munroe, B. Joe, and X. Cheng. (2020). Artificial intelligence and machine learning to fight covid-19. *Physiological Genomics*, 52(4), 200–202. doi: 10.1152/physiolgenomics.00029.2020.
4. Apostolopoulos, I. D., and T. A. Mpesiana. (2020). Covid-19: Automatic detection from X-ray images utilizing transfer learning with convolutional neural networks. *Physical and Engineering Sciences in Medicine*, 43(2), 635–340. doi: 10.1007/s13246-020-00865-4.
5. Stoecklin, S. B. et al. (2020). First cases of coronavirus disease 2019 (COVID-19) in France: Surveillance, investigations and control measures, January 2020. *Eurosurveillance*, 25(6). doi: 10.2807/1560-7917.ES.2020.25.6.2000094.
6. Alqudah, A., S. Qazan, and A. Alqudah. (2020). *Automated Systems for Detection of COVID-19 Using Chest X-ray Images and Lightweight Convolutional Neural Networks*.
7. Choi, W. J., K. N. Lee, E. J. Kang, and H. Lee. (2016). Middle east respiratory syndrome-coronavirus infection: A case report of serial computed tomographic findings in a young male patient. *Korean Journal of Radiology*, 17(1), 166–170. doi: 10.3348/kjr.2016.17.1.166.
8. Chung, M. et al. (2020). CT imaging features of 2019 novel coronavirus (2019-NCoV). *Radiology*, 295(1), 202–207. doi: 10.1148/radiol.2020200230.

9. Fu, S., X. Fu, Y. Song, M. Li, P. Pan, T. Tang, … Y. Ouyang. (2020). Virologic and clinical characteristics for prognosis of severe COVID-19: A retrospective observational study in Wuhan, China. https://doi.org/10.1101/2020.04.03.20051763.
10. Cohen, J. P., P. Morrison, and L. Dao. (2020). COVID-19 image data collection. *GitHub*. https://github.com/ieee8023/covid-chestxray-dataset.
11. He, X. et al. (2020). Sample-efficient deep learning for COVID-19 diagnosis based on CT scans. *Medrxiv*. https://github.com/UCSD-AI4H/COVID-CT.
12. Kermany, D., M. Goldbaum, W. Cai, C. Valentim, H. Liang, S. Baxter, A. McKeown, G. Yang, X. Wu, F. Yan, J. Dong, M. Prasadha, J. Pei, M. Ting, J. Zhu, C. Li, S. Hewett, J. Dong, I. Ziyar, A. Shi, R. Zhang, L. Zheng, R. Hou, W. Shi, X. Fu, Y. Duan, V. Huu, C. Wen, E. Zhang, C. Zhang, O. Li, X. Wang, M. Singer, X. Sun, J. Xu, A. Tafreshi, M. Lewis, H. Xia, and K. Zhang. (2018). Identifying medical diagnoses and treatable diseases by image-based deep learning. *Cell*, 172(5), 1122–1131. doi: 10.1016/j.cell.2018.02.010.
13. Normal CT scans. *Radiopaedia.org*.
14. Dyk, D. A. V., and X. L. Meng. (2001). The art of data augmentation. *Journal of Computational and Graphical Statistics*, 10(1), 1–50. doi: 10.1198/10618600152418584.
15. Shorten, C. and T. M. Khoshgoftaar. (2019). A survey on image data augmentation for deep learning. *Journal of Big Data*, 6, 60. doi: 10.1186/s40537-019-0197-0.
16. Alippi, C., S. Disabato, and M. Roveri. (2018). Moving convolutional neural networks to embedded systems: The AlexNet and VGG-16 Case. In Proceedings of the 17th ACM/IEEE International Conference on Information Processing in Sensor Networks, IPSN 2018. doi: 10.1109/IPSN.2018.00049. AC Med
17. Fu, Sha, Xiaoyu Fu, Yang Song, Min Li, Pin-hua Pan, Tao Tang, Chunhu Zhang, Tiejian Jiang, Deming Tan, Xuegong Fan, Xinping Sha, Jingdong Ma, Yan Huang, Shaling Li, Yixiang Zheng, Zhaoxin Qian, Zeng Xiong, Lizhi Xiao, Huibao Long, and Yi Ouyang. (2020). Virologic and clinical characteristics for prognosis of severe COVID-19: A retrospective observational study in Wuhan, China. 10.1101/2020.04.03.20051763.
18. Kulkarni, S. R., and G. Harman. (2011). Statistical learning theory: A tutorial. *Wiley Interdisciplinary Reviews: Computational Statistics*, 3. doi: 10.1002/wics.179.
19. Clausi, D. A. (2002). An analysis of co-occurrence texture statistics as a function of grey level quantization. *Canadian Journal of Remote Sensing*, 28, 45–62. doi: 10.5589/m02-004.
20. Haralick, R. M., I. Dinstein, and K. Shanmugam. (1973). Textural features for image classification. *IEEE Transactions on Systems, Man and Cybernetics*, 3, 610–621. doi: 10.1109/TSMC.1973.4309314.
21. Soh, L. K., and C. Tsatsoulis. (1999). Texture analysis of SAR sea ice imagery using gray level co-occurrence matrices. *IEEE Transactions on Geoscience and Remote Sensing*, 37, 780–795. doi: 10.1109/36.752194.
22. Thibault, G., J. Angulo, and F. Meyer. (2014). Advanced statistical matrices for texture characterization: Application to cell classification. *IEEE Transactions on Bio-medical Engineering*, 61, 630–637. doi: 10.1109/TBME.2013.2284600.
23. Shensa, M. J. (1992). The discrete wavelet transform: Wedding the à trous and mallat algorithms. *IEEE Transactions on Signal Processing*, 40, 2464–2482. doi: 10.1109/78.157290.
24. Pope, P. E., S. Kolouri, M. Rostami, C. E. Martin, and H. Hoffmann. (2019). Explainability methods for graph convolutional neural networks. In Proceedings of the IEEE Computer Society Conference on Computer Vision and Pattern Recognition. doi: 10.1109/CVPR.2019.01103. IEEE.
25. Selvaraju, R. R., M. Cogswell, A. Das, R. Vedantam, D. Parikh, and D. Batra. (2020). Grad-CAM: Visual explanations from deep networks via gradient-based localization. *International Journal of Computer Vision*, 128, 336–359. doi: 10.1007/s11263-019-01228-7.

4 IoT-Based Micro-Expression Recognition for Nervousness Detection in COVID-Like Condition

Rahul Jain, Vishal Bhardwaj, Vishal Tyagi,
Puneet Singh Lamba, Gopal Chaudhary,
and Fadi Al-Turjman

CONTENTS

4.1 INTRODUCTION

In the last decade, a lot of research has been done in the field of facial expressions using deep learning. A very famous method in deep learning, convolutional neural networks (CNN), is used to solve the facial micro-expressions recognition problem, and we are also going to use it for nervousness detection and other micro-expressions, through video and image [1] extraction. In convolutional neural networks, we can use CNN, recurrent neural network (RNN), or the combinations of both CNN and RNN [2]. As a video contains several separate frames, these technologies can extract special features from each frame. However, there is some limitation with this technology, as it is not able to extract the temporal information from the frame. So, to overcome this limitation, we use 3D CNN models which can extract spatial information and temporal information simultaneously. There is a lot of research in recognizing facial expressions with the help of videos in the area of research. It is difficult to read fake facial expressions, even for humans. It is more difficult for the machines to analyze those. There may be a division in the accuracy because the micro-expressions are dependent on the duration for which the particular expression is carried out on the face. The main components of this research paper are summarized below:

(a) Extracting the spatial and temporal features from the images.
(b) To read out the features of eyes and mouth region and combine the results of both using MicroExpFuseNet.
(c) The intermediate result derived from the above experiments is based upon three-dimensional CNNs.
(d) The effect from the different features is analyzed with the help of salience maps.
(e) 3D CNN kernel sizes also experimented with getting the accurate result of micro-expression recognition.

For a long time, there has been a need to identify human emotions with the help of machines. In this research paper, we are going to analyze facial micro-expressions through video. The need behind facial micro-expression recognition is based on cybercrime and psychological behavior of humans, like nervousness detection. Many unethical organizations use the internet to spread hateful messages in the form of video and to instigate people by showing antisocial things. So, to prevent these hateful messages from videos, we need some software, so that the agenda of these organizations can be abolished. However, some facial expressions cannot be identified by the software, because there is a time constraint. This technology consists of some psychological terms and a computer to recognize facial expressions [3–5].

4.2   RELATED WORK

Hand-designed [6] convolutional neural network method can automatically locate the face [7], then Gabor filters are used for taking out the features. Gabor filters use SVM for recognizing facial expressions [8]. As discussed earlier, the face is divided into sub-parts in which the Gabor filters are applied, and with the help of a 3D gradient orientation histogram descriptor, a correlation is made between all the results. In this way, both micro and macro facial expressions are recognized in any video. Through this, the expressions which are in strain magnitude are also recognized from facial regions like the mouth, forehead, chin, lips, etc. To remove the redundancy in the results, six intersection points technique are used. To get the dynamic texture, a particular technology, LBP [9], i.e. Local Binary Pattern, and three orthogonal planes are used. LBP-TOP [10] lacks the ability to recognize some features, so vector quantization is used to compute the patterns along with codebook, to learn from the resulting patterns.

In today's world, there are high-performing graphics processing units, i.e. GPU-based computers, which make it easy to apply deep learning; datasets having a high number of data learning methods are applied in many sectors, like classification, detection, semantic segmentation [11], etc. Now it is time to apply deep learning in recognizing facial micro-expressions. In this project, SVM and RFC are used to identify micro-expressions by the inclusion of deep and machine learning. CNN uses deep learning to recognize facial expressions where the input is in the form of an image or video. As the face is divided into multiple sub-facial regions, these sub-facial regions are detected via a multi-task convolutional network. For recognizing optical flow [12], fused deep convolutional networks are used. The obtained output is passed into the SVM for recognition and training. There is one drawback of this method, which is that it may lose some temporal information. For training, the micro-expression features can be learned through the expression videos. To consider the minute facial moments, 3D floor-based CNN is used to represent the MFE (Micro face expression) in fine flow [13]. As we have discussed earlier, for the eyes and mouth, MicroExpFuseNet is used, and for the full face, we proposed MicroExpSTCNN. Through the past work, we can easily find out that both the methods give less accuracy and efficiency, but these can be improved with the help of methods inclusive of deep learning-based techniques [14]. That is why we used the 3D CNN method with the inclusion of DL for MER.

4.3 METHODOLOGY

Convolutional neural networks, or CNNs, are extensively used for classification of the image [14], object recognition, and detection. Its structure can be explained in three layers, i.e. pooling, convolution, and classification [15]. Depending upon the application only, we define the architecture of CNN. The factors which define it are the neuron count inside layers, the activation function chosen, and the pooling and convolution layers used.

For image classification, the CNN input is a representation of the image of any color model. In the belief layer, each neuron is linked with the kernel window, which is in turn decorated with images for input during the classification of CNN. This decision kernel [16] comprises the weights of each linked neuron. This determination part produces a series of N images, for each N neuron. These new images may have negative values because of punishment. To resolve this issue, use adjusted linear units (ReLUs) [17] to change negative values with zero values. The output of this layer is called a feature map.

It is common to put the pooling layer right after the convolution layer [17]. This is important, because the pool feature reduces map mobility and reduces network training time. At the end of the call and pooling architecture is a multi-layer perceptron neural network that performs classification based on the feature maps calculated in the previous layers [18]. Due to a large number of layers and successful applications, CNN is a good technique for intensive learning. Its architecture allows automatic extraction of various image attributes such as edges, circles, lines, and textures. Removed attributes further optimize the layer. It is important to emphasize that the kernel filter value applied to the homogeneous layer is the result of back-propagation during CNN training [19–21].

Now, based on the attentional convolutional network, we have proposed the end-to-end deep learning framework [22] which will be used to classify the emotions which underlie the images of the face. In general, if we want to improve the deep neural network, we focus more on the addition of new layers of neurons, sometimes the facilitating flow of gradient, i.e. addition of skip layers, and the more advanced regularization, i.e. spectral normalization, and these things are done when we are doing the problems which involve the classification of larger classes. However, when we are doing facial expression recognition to sense the nervousness in a human or people, which involves classes which are small in number, we use the CNN with attention layers less than ten, which are studied and trained from the beginning and can give the best possible results, as they can surpass the various state-of-the-art products present in different databases. As we can see, in any given face image, all the parts of the face are not important to detect a specific emotion, including nervousness, and in a variety of cases, only particular regions of the face are required to obtain a sense of the possible emotion. Hence, based on our study, we have introduced an attention mechanism, with the help of spatial transformer [23], into our methodology framework, which focuses more on the important regions of the face.

The part of the methodology where feature extraction is present deals with convolution layers which are four in number. After every two layers, there is a maxpooling layer and also a rectified linear unit (ReLU) function, which can be seen in Figure 4.1. After that, there is a dropout layer, and just after that, there is the presence of two fully connected layers. Additionally, there is a spatial transformer, also called the localization [24] network, which consists of the convolution layers

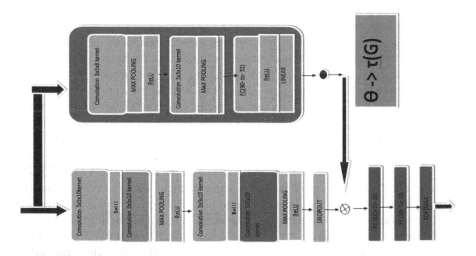

FIGURE 4.1 The proposed model architecture.

(two of them), and these are then, again, followed by the max pooling and ReLU. After the transformation parameters are traversed and operated through, the data to be checked is sent to the sampling grid which produces the warped data. The most relevant parts of the image are focused on by the spatial transformer module, which estimates the sample over the complete attended region [25]. Now, to convert the intake valve to the output, there can be various transformations used, but here we have used an affine transformation, which is used extensively for a lot of applications [26]. The training of the model is carried out by making the optimum result of the loss function with the help of a stochastic gradient descent approach, which is also known as Adam optimizer. The summed-up work of the two, i.e. the classification loss, also called the cross-entropy, and the regularization [27] term, helps in putting up together the loss function. The weight of regularization is set upon the validation set. The addition of dropout and regularization helps us to perfect our model from the beginning irrespective of the size of the dataset, such as JAFFE [28] and CK+ [29]. Here in our work, we have trained different models for every database. Various attempts to increase the accuracy were done, but it didn't help much; for instance, we used more than 40 layers at once. Thus, here we have used the simpler models. Here we have given the full-length explanation of the model we have proposed, focusing on the several facial recognitions in the database. At first, a little something is shown of our model of the work which is used in the database, and then the outputs are compared to various models [30].

4.3.1 ALGORITHM

In this section, we have shown the steps of how we have implemented Micro-Expression Recognition using the attentional Convolutional Neural network. The following steps are done to extract micro-expression using CNN, which is being trained on the Fer2013 [31] Dataset.

Step 1: Preprocessing of data
Step 2: Loading of features and labels into x and y
Step 3: Passing features to train the model and testing using test features
Step 4: Compilation with cross-entropy in the loss function with the help of
    AO, i.e Adam optimizer

In the second step, we are doing a declaration of the required variables. Then, we are assigning seven emotions with labels: 0 is assigned to Angry, 1 to Disgust, 2 to Fear, 3 to Happy, 4 to Sad, 5 to Surprise, and 6 to Neutral. Our input will get processed by batch size of 65. Features are being loaded into two variables, w and z. The third step is the main part of the whole process, as we design CNN where we will pass the features for the training of models and, after that, by testing with features. We are using different CNN-building functions in this project. In the fourth step, the categorical cross-entropy function is used to compile the project using an Adam optimizer. We are using the confusion matrix as the performance parameter.

4.3.2 DATASETS

In this Micro-expression recognition project for nervousness (or negative micro-expression), we are using the FER-2013 [31] dataset. This dataset has about 37,000 high definitions 48×48-pixel grayscale photos of faces. The images are being processed in a way that the faces is well-centered, and every face consists of the same quantity of space in every image. Each of the images has been assigned a category from one of the 7 classes that will show an expression. The image class (a number between 0 and 6) and the given photos are divided into three different sets (training, validation, and test) [32]. There are various images for training to a count of 28,000, out of which there are 3,500 images for validation, 3,500 images for testing, and about 29,000 training images. Every photo in FER-2013 is labeled as one of seven emotions [33]: sad, angry, surprise, happy, disgust, neutral, and afraid, with happiness being the most prevalent expression, providing a baseline. FER-2013 images are made in such a way that they consist of un-posed and posed headshots both, and they are in grayscale [34] and are 48×48 pixels. The gathering of results of Google images found after searching for various emotions and their synonyms helped in creating the FER-2013. So, we shifted our focus to a large extent to the FER-2013 dataset's performance and tried to improve that. As we know, having more images that are un-posed will reflect the images [35]. In Figure 4.2, sample emotions are shown.

4.3.3 PERFORMANCE PARAMETERS

Several parameters can be used for evaluating the execution of the classification and model of machine learning, like confusion matrix, recall score, precision score, F1 score, and ROC curve [36–40].

Recall score: recall score is defined as the score which is the ratio of the correctly predicted values which are positive to all observations in the actual class.

F1 score: the average is taken of the recall, and the precision can be called the F1 score, and therefore, it has both positive and negative values.

Precision score: this can be defined as the ratio of the correctly predicted positive values to the total predicted positive values.

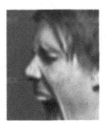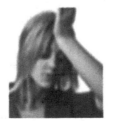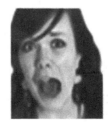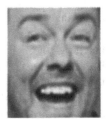

FIGURE 4.2   Four sample images from FER dataset.

ROC curve: (Receiver Operating Characteristics curve) is another parameter metric to calculate the performance in the classifier model. The ROC curve shows the locus of rates of true positives with the rate of false positives. The ideal classifier will have a ROC where the graph will show a true positive rate of a hundred percent with zero development of the x-axis, i.e., false positive. The performance of a classifier is described with the help of a **Confusion Matrix**, which is easy to understand because it is in a tabular form that operates on a set of data for which the true values are already known.

4.4 EXPERIMENTAL RESULTS

The comparison of results concerning the accuracy of MicroExpStCnn and MicroExpFuseNet, with the results of the state methods, deep learning methods, and the reported accuracies of handcrafted methods for micro-expression recognition are listed in Table 4.1:

We have analyzed the images from Fer2013 databases. The raw performance of CNN [47] is shown in Table 4.2.

TABLE 4.1
Score Comparison between Different Algorithms [41–46]

Algorithms	SCORE
LBP-TOP	0.42
STCLQP	0.64
CNN with Augmentation	0.78
3D-FCNN	0.55
MicroEXPSTCNN	0.68
MicroExpFUSENET (Intermediate)	0.82
Attentional Neural Network	0.67

TABLE 4.2
Performance Parameters

Mood	Precision Score	Recall Score	F1 Score	Support Score
Neutral	0.96	0.76	0.85	2565
Positive	0.29	0.92	0.44	62
Negative	0.38	0.80	0.52	422
Surprise	0.87	0.58	0.70	112
Average	0.87	0.76	0.79	3161

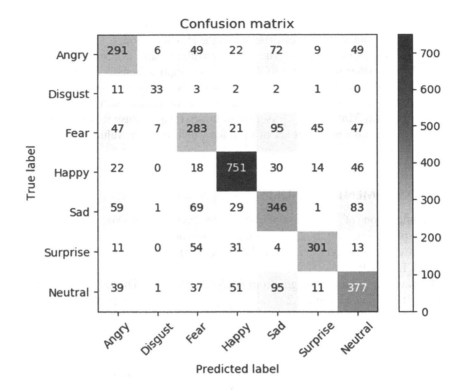

FIGURE 4.3   Confusion matrix resulting from FER2013 dataset.

It can be easily analyzed from Figure 4.3, which shows the confusion Matrix, that most of the confusions are present between neutral negative and surprise neutral classes. This is due to the movement of eyebrows and blinking of eyes.

4.4.1   ACCURACY

The accuracy of this MER, i.e micro-expression recognition and nervousness detection model, is **67%**. This project can easily identify the negative and sad expressions of the patients. The right treatment can then be given to the patient on time to reduce the chance of suicide.

4.5   CONCLUSION

COVID-19 is an unprecedented event, and tackling this pandemic is a challenging task, but a technologically driven telemedicine field can fight this situation, so we have proposed two 3-Dimensional CNNs for Facial micro-expression recognition from videos recorded while conferencing with doctors online. We have used 3D Convolutional Neural Network for the shared convolutions in temporal and spatial directions which cause the occurring spatio-temporal training. Our diligent experiments on CNNs over the standard dataset manifest that, other than the mouth and eye area, some prominent facial areas can provide facial micro-expression recognition. We have also analyzed the 3-dimensional kernel, and we found that deep temporal and small spatial filters work better. In the upcoming time, we will surely be able to extend this work by multiple experiments on different areas of the face, and will be able to analyze the main facial regions for facial micro-expression recognition. For detecting facial micro-expressions, attention plays an important role, which makes our model capable of recognizing emotions with less than 10 layers of performance. We have also compared with other famous facial expression recognition databases, along with providing favorable results. Visualization methods are also used to highlight the important areas of the face, which ultimately helps in giving subsequently accurate and acceptable results.

REFERENCES

1. Ekman, P. (2009). Lie catching and microexpressions. *The Philosophy of Deception*, 1(2), 5.
2. Takalkar, M., M. Xu, Q. Wu, and Z. Chaczko. (2018). A survey: Facial micro-expression recognition. *Multimedia Tools and Applications*, 77(15), 19301–19325.
3. Al-hababi, M. M. Khan, F. Al-Turjman, N. Zhao, and X. Yang. (2020). Ubiquitous intelligent edge computing testbed for post-surgery monitoring by machine learning algorithms. *Journal of Cloud Computing*.
4. Ullah, Z., F. Al-Turjman, L. Mostarda, and R. Gagliardi. (2020). Applications of artificial intelligence and machine learning in smart cities. *Elsevier Computer Communications Journal*, 154, 313–323.
5. Al-Turjman, Fadi, and Ilyes Baali. "Machine learning for wearable IoT-based applications: A survey." *Transactions on Emerging Telecommunications Technologies* (2019): e3635.
6. Mukherjee, S., B. Vamshi, K. S. V. K. Reddy, R. V. Krishna, and S. V. S. Harish. (2016). Recognizing facial expressions using novel motion based features. In Proceedings of the 10th Indian Conference on Computer Vision, Graphics and Image Processing (pp. 1–8). AC Med
7. Li, X., X. Hong, A. Moilanen, X. Huang, T. Pfister, G. Zhao, and M. Pietikäinen. (2017). Towards reading hidden emotions: A comparative study of spontaneous micro-expression spotting and recognition methods. *IEEE Transactions on Affective Computing*, 9(4), 563–577.
8. Merghani, Walied, Adrian K. Davison, and Moi Hoon Yap. "A review on facial micro-expressions analysis: datasets, features and metrics." *arXiv preprint arXiv:1805.02397* (2018).
9. Huang, X., S.-J. Wang, G. Zhao, and M. Pietikainen. (2015). Facial micro-expression recognition using spatiotemporal local binary pattern with integral projection. In Proceedings of the IEEE International Conference on Computer Vision Workshops (pp. 1–9). IEEE.
10. Wang, Y., J. See, R. C-W. Phan, and Y.-H. Oh. (2014). Lbp with six intersection points: Reducing redundant information in lbp-top for micro-expression recognition. In Asian Conference on Computer Vision (pp. 525–537). Springer.
11. Goodfellow, I., Y. Bengio, and A. Courville. (2016). *Deep Learning*. MIT Press.
12. Krizhevsky, Alex, Ilya Sutskever, and Geoffrey E. Hinton. "Imagenet classification with deep convolutional neural networks." In *Advances in neural information processing systems*, pp. 1097–1105. 2012..

13. Vishal D., B. Takkar, and P. S. Lamba. (2020). Micro-expression recognition using 3D – CNN. *Fusion: Practice and Applications*, 1(1), 5–13. DOI: 10.5281/zenodo. 3825862.

14. Liu, Y.-J., J.-K. Zhang, W.-J. Yan, S.-J. Wang, G. Zhao, and X. Fu. (2015). A main directional mean optical flow feature for spontaneous micro-expression recognition. *IEEE Transactions on Affective Computing*, 7(4), 299–310.

15. Hou, W., X. Gao, D. Tao, and X. Li. (2014). Blind image quality assessment via deep learning. *IEEE Transactions on Neural Networks and Learning Systems*, 26(6), 1275–1286.

16. Nagpal, C., and S. R. Dubey. (2019). A performance evaluation of convolutional neural networks for face anti-spoofing. In 2019 International Joint Conference on Neural Networks (IJCNN) (pp. 1–8). IEEE.

17. Minaee, S., and A. Abdolrashidi. (2019). Deep-emotion: Facial expression recognition using attentional convolutional network. arXiv:1902.01019.

18. Guo, J., S. Zhou, J. Wu, J. Wan, X. Zhu, Z. Lei, and S. Z. Li. (2017). Multi-modality network with visual and geometrical information for micro emotion recognition. In 2017 12th IEEE International Conference on Automatic Face & Gesture Recognition (FG 2017) (pp. 814–819). IEEE.

19. Jacob, S., V. Menon, F. Al-Turjman, P. G. Vinoj, and L. Mostarda. (2019). Artificial muscle intelligence system with deep learning for post-stroke assistance and rehabilitation. *IEEE Access*, 7(1), 133463–133473.

20. Serte, Sertan, Ali Serener, and Fadi Al-Turjman. "Deep learning in medical imaging: A brief review." *Transactions on Emerging Telecommunications Technologies* (2020): e4080 1–14.

21. Al-Turjman, F., U. Ulusar, and M. Nawaz. (2020). Intelligence in the internet of medical things era: A systematic review of current and future trends. *Elsevier Computer Communications Journal*, 150(15), 644–660.

22. Gan, Y. S., S.-T. Liong, W.-C. Yau, Y.-C. Huang, and L.-K. Tan. (2019). Off-apexnet on micro-expression recognition system. *Signal Processing: Image Communication*, 74, 129–139.

23. Jaderberg, Max, Karen Simonyan, and Andrew Zisserman. "Spatial transformer networks." In *Advances in neural information processing systems*, pp. 2017–2025. 2015.

24. Patel, D., X. Hong, and G. Zhao. (2016). Selective deep features for micro-expression recognition. In 2016 23rd International Conference on Pattern Recognition (ICPR) (pp. 2258–2263). IEEE.

25. Wu, Q., X. Shen, and X. Fu. (2011). The machine knows what you are hiding: An automatic micro-expression recognition system. In International Conference on Affective Computing and Intelligent Interaction (pp. 152–162). Springer.

26. Polikovsky, S., Y. Kameda, and Y. Ohta. Facial micro-expressions recognition using a high-speed camera and 3D-gradient descriptor. In 3rd International Conference on Imaging for Crime Detection and Prevention (ICDP 2009) (p. 16).

27. Lu, H., K. Kpalma, and J. Ronsin. (2018). Motion descriptors for micro-expression recognition. *Signal Processing: Image Communication*, 67, 108–117.

28. Lyons, M. J., S. Akamatsu, M. Kamachi, J. Gyoba, and J. Budynek. (1998). The Japanese female facial expression (JAFFE) database. In 3rd International Conference on Automatic Face and Gesture Recognition (pp. 14–16).

29. Lucey, P., J. F. Cohn, T. Kanade, J. Saragih, Z. Ambadar, and I. Matthews. The extended cohn-kanade dataset (ck+): A complete dataset for action unit and emotion-specified expression. In 2010 IEEE Computer Society Conference on Computer Vision and Pattern Recognition-Workshops (pp. 94–101). IEEE.

30. Zhao, G., and M. Pietikainen. (2007). Dynamic texture recognition using local binary patterns with an application to facial expressions. IEEE Transactions on Pattern Analysis and Machine Intelligence 29(6), 915–928.

31. Giannopoulos, P., I. Perikos, and I. Hastily Geroudis. (2018). Deep learning approaches for facial emotion recognition: A case study on FER-2013. In *Advances in Hybridization of Intelligent Methods* (pp. 1–16). Springer.

32. Huang, X., G. Zhao, X. Hong, W. Zheng, and M. Pietikäinen. Spontaneous facial micro-expression analysis using spatiotemporal completed local quantized patterns. *Neurocomputing*, 175, 564–578.

33. Grobova, J., M. Colovic, M. Marjanovic, A. Njegus, H. Demire, and G. Anbarjafari. (2017). Automatic hidden sadness detection using micro-expressions. In 2017 12th IEEE International Conference on Automatic Face & Gesture Recognition (FG 2017) (pp. 828–832). IEEE.

34. Li, X., J. Yu, and S. Zhan. (2016). Spontaneous facial micro-expression detection based on deep learning. In 2016 IEEE 13th International Conference on Signal Processing (ICSP) (pp. 1130–1134). IEEE.

35. M. Takalkar, and M. Xu. (2017). Image based facial micro-expression recognition using deep learning on small datasets. In International Conference on Digital Image Computing: Techniques and Applications (DICTA). IEEE.

36. Goutte, C., and E. Gaussier. (2005). A probabilistic interpretation of precision, recall and F-score, with implication for evaluation. In European Conference on Information Retrieval (pp. 345–359). Springer.

37. Huang, H., H. Xu, X. Wang, and W. Silamu. (2015). Maximum F1-score discriminative training criterion for automatic mispronunciation detection. *IEEE/ACM Transactions on Audio, Speech, and Language Processing*, 23(4), 787–797.

38. Mellenbergh, G. J. (1996). Measurement precision in test score and item response models. *Psychological Methods*, 1(3), 293.

39. Visa, S., B. Ramsay, A. L. Ralescu, and E. Van Der Knaap. (2011). Confusion matrix-based feature selection. *MAICS*, 710, 120–127.

40. Hajian-Tilaki, K. (2013). Receiver operating characteristic (ROC) curve analysis for medical diagnostic test evaluation. *Caspian Journal of Internal Medicine*, 4(2), 627.

41. X. Li, T. Pfister, X. Huang, G. Zhao, and M. Pietikainen. (2013). A spontaneous micro-expression database: Inducement, collection and baseline, In 10th IEEE International Conference And Workshops on Automatic Face and Gesture Recognition (fg), 2013 (pp. 1–6). IEEE.

42. Huang, X., G. Zhao, X. Hong, W. Zheng, and M. Pietikäinen. (2016). Spontaneous facial micro-expression analysis using spatiotemporal completed local quantized patterns. *Neurocomputing*, 175, 564–578.

43. Takalkar, M., and M. Xu. (2017). Image based facial micro-expression recognition using deep learning on small datasets. In International Conference on Digital Image Computing: Techniques and Applications (DICTA). IEEE.

44. Li, J., Y. Wang, J. See, and W. Liu. (2019). Micro-expression recognition based on 3D flow convolutional neural network. *Pattern Analysis and Applications*, 22(4), 1331–1339.

45. Reddy, S. P. T., S. T. Karri, S. R. Dubey, and S. Mukherjee. (2019). Spontaneous facial micro-expression recognition using 3D spatio temporal convolutional neural networks. In 2019 International Joint Conference on Neural Networks (IJCNN) (pp. 1–8). IEEE.

46. Song, B., K. Li, Y. Zong, J. Zhu, W. Zheng, J. Shi, and L. Zhao. (2019). Recognizing spontaneous micro-expression using a three-stream convolutional neural network. *IEEE Access*, 7, 184537–184551.

47. Borza, Diana, Razvan Itu, and Radu Danescu. "Micro Expression Detection and Recognition from High Speed Cameras using Convolutional Neural Networks." In *VISIGRAPP (5: VISAPP)*, pp. 201–208. 2018.

5 Genetically Optimized Computer-Aided Diagnosis for Detection and Classification of COVID-19

S. Punitha, Fadi Al-Turjman, and Thompson Stephan

CONTENTS

5.1   INTRODUCTION

Coronavirus disease 2019 (COVID-19) was first identified amid an outbreak of respiratory illness cases in Wuhan City, Hubei Province, China. It is defined as an illness caused by a novel coronavirus now called severe acute respiratory syndrome coronavirus 2 (SARS-CoV-2; formerly called 2019-nCoV). The COVID-19 epidemic was declared a public health emergency by the World Health Organization (WHO) on 30 January 2020. This virus has led to a rapid increase in the number of people being affected. As of 9 May 2020, a total of 3,855,788 confirmed Coronavirus cases globally, with 265,862 deaths [1] had been reported by WHO. Easily available imaging equipment, like thoracic CT and chest X-ray, are used to identify COVID-19 and are highly helpful in clinical practice [2–5]. Another study looked at clinical characteristics in COVID-19 positively tested close contacts of COVID-19 patients [6]. Approximately 30% of those COVID-19-positive close contacts never developed any symptoms or changes on chest CT scans. The remainder showed changes in CT, but ~20% reportedly developed symptoms during their hospital course, and none of them developed severe disease [6]. Considering the number of COVID-19 cases increasing day by day, an enhanced diagnosis is required to eliminate the need for multiple diagnoses. Also, this viral exposure is making healthcare practitioners susceptible. Therefore, this dangerous viral transmission can be constrained through proper analysis of the image findings. Generally, the CT images are processed in three successive stages starting with pre-scan preparation, followed by image acquisition, and finally disease diagnosis.

Recently, COVID-19 cases are diagnosed using emerging medical imaging technologies, importantly Artificial intelligence (AI) [7], which ensures more safety, accuracy, and reliability. The importance of imaging for COVID-19 detection [8] is also highlighted in the recent Chinese diagnosis and treatment protocol for COVID-19 (trial version 7). The mild, moderate, severe, or critically ill cases are the major classifications of the confirmed COVID-19 cases analyzed, based on the chest imaging. A comprehensive review [9] of imaging data acquisition, segmentation, and diagnosis for COVID-19 are much needed to discover the opportunities of using AI techniques [10] for diagnosing this disease. The deep learning technology-inspired AI techniques were highly successful in medical imaging, owing to its ability to properly extract features [11]. More importantly, the bacterial and viral pneumonia in pediatric chest radiographs was detected and differentiated using deep learning models [12]. Moreover, several studies were conducted for detecting different imaging features of chest CT [13]. Recent times have seen several models being developed for the successful integration of AI techniques to battle COVID-19 cases. These techniques have a high scope of progression in the field of real-time medical imaging applications and could stop this current epidemic.

5.2   RELATED WORKS

Li et al. [14] identified COVID-19 on chest CT exams using a deep learning method. This deep learning model was used for accurate detection and differentiation from community-acquired pneumonia and other lung diseases. The developed fully automatic framework [14] to detect COVID-19 was tested over a collected dataset consisting of 4,356 chest CT exams from 3,322 patients. Ozturk et al. [15] performed an automatic diagnosis of COVID-19 using a deep learning model. This model doesn't use any feature extraction methods and displays an end-to-end architecture and performs diagnosis without the use of raw chest X-ray images. Narin et al. [16] proposed a deep convolution neural network technique for automatic prediction of COVID-19. This model uses chest X-ray images and pre-trained transfer models.

Apostolopoulos et al. [17] studied and evaluated the performance of various convolutional neural network (CNN) architectures proposed over the recent years for classifying medical images. One of the best methods for pneumonia chest diagnosis is Computed Tomography (CT) scanning. Importantly, the hospitals are using CT images of the chest to early-classify COVID-19 patients. However, classification based on CT images requires significant time and the expertise of radiologists. Thus, frontline clinical doctors need to have promising automated diagnosis and analysis techniques to cope with the increasing COVID-19 infection rate and save critical time for disease control. Concerning CT image analysis, efficient AI techniques are needed, as the classification process is difficult, owing to a greater number of variable objects, since some irrelevant areas outside the lungs are included during diagnosis.

Gozes et al. [18] distinguished patients with coronavirus using AI-based automated CT image analysis tools for coronavirus detection and monitoring. Singh et al. [19] proposed a multi-objective, differential, evolution-based CNN for classifying chest CT images of COVID-19 patients. This work uses multi-objective differential evolution (MODE),which is used to tune the initial parameters of CNN. Shan et al. [20] proposed a deep learning technique on the chest CT scans to automatically segment and quantify the infected regions and the complete lung region. This proposed technique used 249 COVID-19 patients' CT images for training and 300 new COVID-19 patients' CT images for validation. To filter the automatic annotation of each COVID-19 case, a human-in-the-loop (HITL) strategy was adopted to assist the radiologists. The authors [20] quantitatively evaluated the accuracy of their proposed technique to automatically delineate the infected regions. Xu et al. [21] proposed and applied a deep learning technique on 618 pulmonary CT image samples for distinguishing COVID-19 pneumonia from Influenza-A viral pneumonia and other unrelated cases. The confidence score and the type of infection for a particular CT case were computed using Noisy-or Bayesian function. Wang et al. [22] made use of the advantage of the radiographical changes in 453 COVID-19 CT images and used an AI-based deep learning technique for extracting the COVID-19 features. Sethy et al. [23] proposed a technique for detecting coronavirus-infected patients using X-ray images and the use of the deep learning-based methods. The coronavirus-affected X-ray images were classified using the support vector machine (SVM) classifier.

5.3 PROBLEM DEFINITION

In existing works, identification of COVID-19 has been carried out using data acquisition and with the help of interface systems. Techniques that detect the infected portions of lung have been proposed for successful segmentation of the infected portions. To design an effective automatic diagnostic system for COVID-19 is the main challenge for us. From the existing techniques studied, not many researchers have classified the different severity levels such as pneumonia, COVID-19 pneumonia, and other infections based on the CT scan lung images. Sensitivity and specificity levels of some of the CAD techniques designed for COVID-19 are high in the literature. When CT lung images are considered, the segmentation is challenging, and lungs and the thorax areas are extracted. In the case of the infected portions of the lungs, the intensity and the texture features vary when compared to the non-infected portions. This difference can be used to detect the infected portions. Most existing methodologies used to detect COVID-19 are complex.

5.4 PROPOSED METHODOLOGY

The proposed methodology deals with the identification of the infected portions in a lung CT scan image and classifies them as pneumonia, COVID-pneumonia, and other infections. The proposed methodology uses the image processing techniques: pre-processing, Region of Interest (ROI) segmentation, and classification, as shown in Figure 5.1. The statistical and wavelet features are derived from the lung CT scan image. The statistical features extracted are mean, area, skewness, and wavelet feature using Discrete Wavelet transform (DWT).

After feature extraction, an ANN model based on an optimized fuzzy classifier is used for classifying the CT lung images as normal or abnormal. Further, a genetically optimized region growing algorithm is used to extract the infected portions from the abnormal images. Then the texture and intensity features are extracted from the segmented portions and fed as input to an optimized ANN model that is trained using the backpropagation algorithm. The optimized ANN model is then used to classify the segmented portions as pneumonia, COVID-pneumonia, and other infections. The optimized neural network is generated where the initial weights, hidden weights, and learning rates are optimized using a genetic algorithm. With the help of the proposed approach, COVID-19 can effectively be detected and diagnosed in the early stages. The performance of the proposed method is analyzed using True Positive, True Negative, False Positive, False Negative, and accuracy. This can be compared with existing techniques. The proposed method can be implemented using MATLAB and can be evaluated with the help of publicly available datasets.

5.4.1 DATA ACQUISITION

The proposed methodology uses lung CT scan images that are abnormal and contain infectious regions that are affected by COVID-19 pneumonia, normal pneumonia, and other infections. The images are collected from a publicly available dataset [24] that contains a total of 471 CT lung images. This dataset contains 275 CT scan images of COVID-19 and 195 CT images of non-COVID-19(normal and other infections). These images are used by the proposed methodology for segmentation and classification purposes. The sample images from the dataset are shown in Figure 5.2.

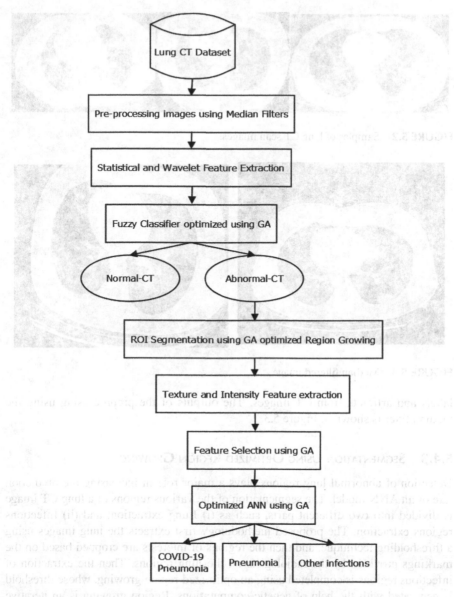

FIGURE 5.1 The Proposed architecture for detection and classification of lung CT images.

5.4.2 PREPROCESSING

The preprocessing of lung CT images is done using 3×3 median filters in which a 3×3 window is utilized, and output values are calculated by taking the median of neighboring pixels. These filters help to eliminate the Gaussian, salt, and pepper noise in the lung regions. The thresholding techniques can be involved to remove

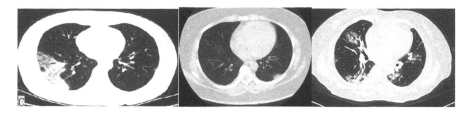

FIGURE 5.2   Samples of lung CT scan images.

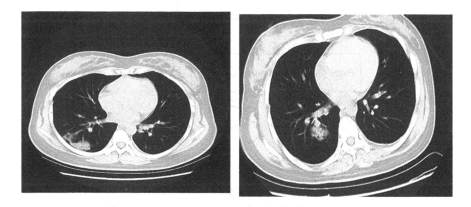

FIGURE 5.3   Median filtered image.

labels and artifacts from CT images. The outputs of the preprocessing using the median filter is shown in Figure 5.3.

5.4.3   SEGMENTATION USING OPTIMIZED REGION GROWING

Detection of abnormal lung regions plays a major role in increasing the prediction rate of an ANN model. The segmentation of the various regions of a lung CT image is divided into two different parts, such as (i) Lung extraction; and (ii) Infections regions extraction. The proposed methodology first extracts the lung images using a thresholding technique, and then the regions of interests are cropped based on the markings provided by the radiologists on the lung regions. Then the extraction of infectious regions is completed using an optimized region growing, whose threshold is generated with the help of genetic computations. Region growing is an iterative approach for pixel classification that uses a set of initial seeds in which the neighboring pixels are checked and iteratively aggregated based on different similarity constraints. Traditional region growing uses a static threshold for aggregation of similar pixels. Since the intensity of the infected portions varies, the proposed work uses a dynamic optimized threshold that is generated using genetic operations that vary in each iteration. The proposed work greatly segments the infected regions from the abnormal lung CT images, making segmentation more accurate. The infected regions are further classified as pneumonia, COVID-pneumonia, and other infections. The extraction of the lungs and the infectious regions are shown in the Figures 5.4 and 5.5.

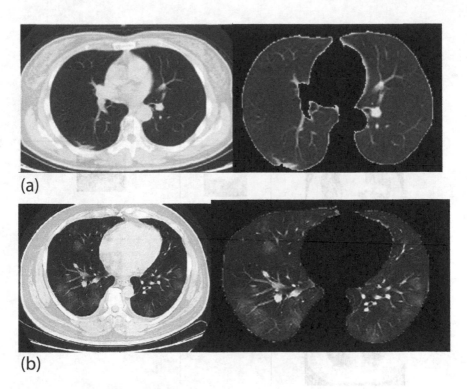

FIGURE 5.4   (a) Filtered image (b) Lung extraction.

5.4.4 Feature Extraction and Feature Selection

The classification accuracy depends on extracted features and features that are selected that correctly identify and classify the infected regions. The proposed work extracts the statistical feature and wavelet features during the first stage of classification. The statistical features are intensity, skewness, and texture features. The texture features extracted using the local Gabor XOR pattern (LGXP) and discrete wavelet transform (DWT) is used to extract the wavelet features at the first stage classification. In the second stage classification, the texture features are extracted using the gray level co-occurrence matrix (GLCM), and intensity features based on the histogram are extracted. Then the significant features are selected using a feature selection process optimized using a GA algorithm that forms as the input to an optimized ANN model. Table 5.1 shows the features that are extracted from the infected regions.

5.4.5 Two Stage Classification Using Genetically Optimized ANN Classification

The proposed approach utilizes a two-stage classification where the first stage classifies the lung CT images as normal and abnormal using an optimized fuzzy classifier and the second stage is processed on abnormal images and classifies based on the

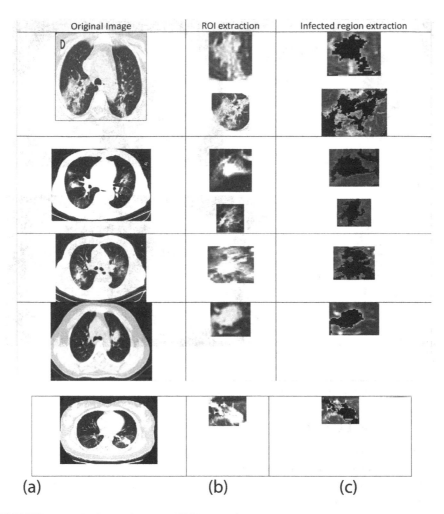

FIGURE 5.5 (a) Filtered image (b) ROI extraction (c) Infected region extraction.

TABLE 5.1
Texture and Intensity Features Extracted from Infectious Regions

Feature Labels	Feature Name
Intensity Histogram features (f1, f2, f3, f4, f5)	Mean, Variance, Skewness, Kurtosis, Entropy
Texture features (f6, f7, f8, f9, f10, f11, f12, f13, f14, f15, f16, f17, f18, f19, f20)	Energy, Contrast, Cluster prominence, Dissimilarity, Correlation, Entropy, Sum of squares, Information measure of correlation, Homogeneity, Maximum probability,Long runs emphasis, Short runs emphasis, Gray level non-uniformity, Run length non-uniformity, Run percentage

severity in the infected regions of pneumonia, COVID-pneumonia, and other infections. This section describes the two-stage classification in detail.

5.4.5.1 Stage 1 Classification

The first stage of classification in the proposed work consists of the fuzzy classifier which is optimized using genetic operations like initialization of chromosomes, fitness function evaluation, mutation operations, crossover operations, and optimal selection. The classification uses a GA optimized fuzzy classifier, where the optimal fuzzy rules are generated and used for classification as normal and abnormal CT lung image. The GA uses input features based on statistical and wavelet features and generates the optimal rule set that is stored in the rule base of the fuzzy classifier. With the help of membership functions and optimal fuzzy rules, the fuzzy classifier groups images in the training phase as normal and abnormal, and in the testing phase, fuzzified input and rules are matched, and the appropriate fuzzy score is calculated. Thus, the first stage fuzzy classifier consists of the fuzzy rule set generated using genetic algorithm, membership function, and classification of lung CT images collected using data acquisition. The samples of the normal and abnormal lung CT images collected from the dataset are shown in Figures 5.6. The optimized fuzzy classifier is shown in Figure 5.7.

5.4.5.2 Stage 2 Classification

The proposed methodology uses Feed-Forward neural network (FFNN), whose initial weights, hidden nodes, and learning rate is optimized using GA for accurate classification of lung CT images of pneumonia, COVID-pneumonia, and other infections. The basic process involved is proposed to be genetically optimized ANN, which is explained in Algorithm 1.The optimized selection of individual chromosomes is used for the generation of initial weights and hidden nodes of ANN that is trained using a backpropagation algorithm achieving local minima. The classifier is trained using the trained dataset collected from publicly available lung COVID-19–affected CT images. The training used is the Levenberg-Marquardt backpropagation algorithm where the learning rate, momentum, termination criteria, number

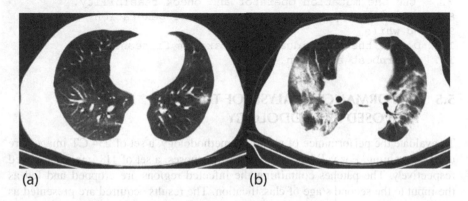

(a)   (b)

FIGURE 5.6   (a) Normal (b) Abnormal.

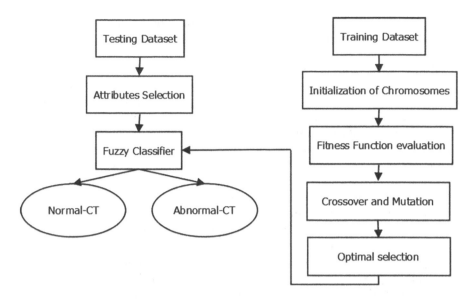

FIGURE 5.7   Genetically optimized fuzzy classification.

of input neurons, hidden layers, hidden neurons, and the output neurons are the parameters used.

Algorithm 1: Genetic Algorithm
Input: Parameter *pop_size*.
Output: The best individual in all generations
1. Choose encode method.
2. Perform Initialization of *pop_size* individuals.
3. *while*i<*Maximum_iteration* and *Best_fitness<Maximum_fitness*do
4.   Calculate Fitness of each individual.
5.   Perform Selection process.
6.   Use the crossover operator and check feasibility.
7.   Use the mutation operator and check feasibility.
8.   Update the population for the next generation.
9. *end while*
10. Decode the individual with maximum fitness.
11. *return*best solution.

5.5   PERFORMANCE ANALYSIS OF THE PROPOSED METHODOLOGY

To evaluate the performance of proposed methodology, a set of 234 CT images are used for training. For validation and testing purposes, a set of 118 images are used respectively. The patches containing the infected regions are cropped and fed as the input to the second stage of classification. The results acquired are presented as segmentation and classification performance for the proposed ABCNN approach.

TABLE 5.2

Parameter Settings of the Proposed Approach

Parameter	Value
Training	Back propagation
Input nodes size	20
Output nodes size	2
Initial weights (Number of bits)	15
Hidden node size (Number of bits)	2
Input features (Number of bits)	20
Activation function (hidden node)	Hyperbolic tangent
Activation function (output node)	Pure linear
Training set (no of samples)	234 (50%)
Validation set (no of samples)	118 (25%)
Testing set (no of samples)	118 (25%)
Population size	80
Crossover percentage	0.8
Mutation percentage	0.5
Mutation rate	0.02
Chromosome selection	Roulette wheel method

5.5.1 PARAMETER SETTINGS AND EXPERIMENTAL SETUP

The proposed methodology is implemented using MATLAB (software MATLAB version R2019a) using a PC with characteristics: Intel Pentium i5 8th gen processor, 8 GB of RAM and windows-10 operating system. The neural network toolbox is used for backpropagation training. The training parameters for the implementation of backpropagation isdefault. The winner-take-all approach is used for classification at output nodes. The parameter settings of the proposed method are shown in Table 5.2.

5.5.2 SEGMENTATION PERFORMANCE OF PROPOSED METHODOLOGY

Accuracy based on segmentation results indicates the eventual success or failure of the segmentation process. To evaluate the performance of segmentation of the proposed ABCNN approach, DICE and Jaccard are used. DICE represents the degree of overlapping between two binary images, and Jaccard indicates the degree of similarity. These are defined using Equation (1 and 2) in which X and Y indicate the manually segmented infected regions and output image of the optimized region growing segmentation method, respectively.

$$\text{DICE}(X,Y) = \frac{2|X \cap Y|}{|X| + |Y|} \tag{5.1}$$

$$\text{Jaccard} = \frac{|X \cap Y|}{|X \cup Y|} \qquad (5.2)$$

The segmentation results of the proposed approach are shown in Table 5.3.

5.5.3 CLASSIFICATION PERFORMANCE OF THE PROPOSED APPROACH

The proposed methodology for diagnosing the COVID-19 disease is evaluated as the means of sensitivity, specificity, and accuracy with the help of True positive True Negative, False Positive and False Negative values. The proposed methodology is computed for generation sizes 10, 20 and 30, as shown in Table 5.4.Significant changes in the level of accuracy and complexity has been noted for different back-propagation algorithms, like resilient back propagation, Levenberg Marquardt, and momentum-based gradient decent. The main aim of the proposed approach is to build an ANN network with optimal input feature set, initial weights, and hidden node size with less network error, complexity, and computational time. The convergence of classification accuracy and number of connections is shown in Figures 5.8 and 5.9.

The proposed methodology, with respect to RP, achieved the highest classification accuracy (mean) of 89.37% for ten independent runs at a generation size of 20. Followed by GD, whichachieved a high accuracy of85.59% at 30thgeneration size. Next to GD, LM achieved 88.13% at 30thgeneration size. The accuracy of RP is 4.53% more than LM and 1.41% more than GD. The number of connections (average) for RP is 18.25 at 20th generation size. Followed by RP, GD produced 19.95 mean connections at 30th generation size. Next to GD, LM produced 20.21 mean connections at 30th generation size. RP has generated less complex ANN compared to the other two variants. RP achieved a complexity of 8.5% less than GD and 9.7% less than LM.

The confusion matrix in Table 5.5 shows the classification performance of the proposed approach. A total number of 800 COVID-19cases and 380non-COVID-19 cases were investigated for ten independent runs. True Positive (TP), True Negative (TN), False Positive (FP), and False Negative (FN) were calculated.

TABLE 5.3

Segmentation Results of the Proposed Approach

Segmented portions	DICE (%)	Jaccard (%)
	0.86	0.83
	0.84	0.81

TABLE 5.4
Performance Evaluation of the Proposed ABCNN Approach

Max Generation Size	RP				LM				GD			
	Classification Accuracy (%)		Number of Connections		Classification Accuracy (%)		Number of Connections		Classification Accuracy (%)		Number of Connections	
	Best	Mean	Best	Mean	Best	Mean	Best	Mean	Best	Mean	Best	Mean
10	85.31	83.25	21	22.65	82.21	81.22	24	25.52	86.95	87.02	22	23.65
20	90.60	89.83	17	18.25	84.33	83.58	20	21.34	87.60	86.65	20	21.15
30	89.12	88.92	19	19.26	86.03	85.59	19	20.21	89.12	88.13	18	19.95

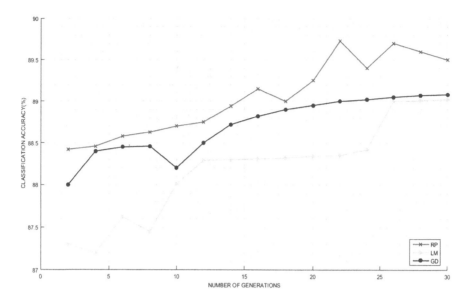

FIGURE 5.8   Performance in terms of classification accuracy.

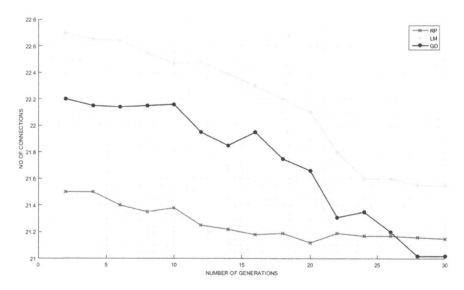

FIGURE 5.9   Evolution of number of connections for different generations.

The performance metrics of the proposed approach in terms of sensitivity, specificity, and other measures are listed in Table 5.6. The sensitivity and specificity are high for RP compared to GD and LM. Table 5.7 shows the confusion matrix for the best network obtained by RP with optimal selected input features.

The classifier performance of the proposed methodology in terms of the average computational time is shown in Table 5.8. The average computational time is noted

TABLE 5.5
Confusion Matrix of the Proposed Approach for Ten Runs

Methods of Comparison	Actual	Number of Cases	Test Outcome-Predicted COVID	Non-COVID
RP	COVID	800	735(TP)	55(FN)
	Non-COVID	380	65(FP)	325(TN)
LM	COVID	800	705 (TP)	75(FN)
	Non-COVID	380	95(FP)	305 (TN)
GD	COVID	800	720(TP)	60(FN)
	Non-COVID	380	80(FP)	320(TN)

TABLE 5.6
Performance Based on Different Metrics

Metrics	RP	LM	GD
Sensitivity (%)	93.03	90.38	92.30
Specificity (%)	83.33	76.25	83.75
Accuracy (%)	89.83	85.59	88.13
Precision(%)	91.8	88.1	90
Negative predictive Value (NPV) (%)	85.52	80.26	84.21
F measure	0.9245	0.8924	0.9113

TABLE 5.7
Confusion Matrix with Selected Features

Feature Selection	Actual Cases		Predicted Cases Benign	Malignant	Selected Feature Set
With Feature	COVID	80	75(TP)	6(FN)	f2, f3, f8, f9, f12, f14, f16,
Selection	Non-COVID	38	5(FP)	32(TN)	f17, f19
Without Feature	COVID	80	68(TP)	13(FN)	Total dataset from
Selection	Non-COVID	38	12(FP)	25(TN)	Table 5.1

for ten independent runs at generation sizes 10, 20, and 30. The LM requires less computational time, followed by RP and GD.

Figure 5.10 shows a comparison of the proposed approach with other evolutionary algorithms, like Particle Swarm Optimization (PSO), Differential Evolution (DE), and Dragonfly Algorithm (DA). The aforementioned algorithms are executed with

TABLE 5.8

Performance Based on Computational Time

Maximum Generation Size	Average CPU Time(s)		
	RP	LM	GD
10	555.3	532.5	640.2
20	789.6	720.6	805.9
30	1000.7	954.8	1076.1

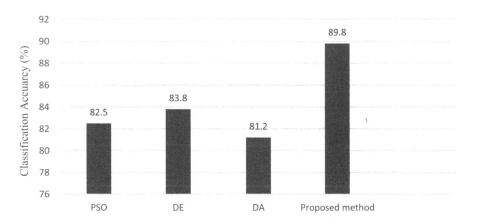

FIGURE 5.10   Comparison with other evolutionary methods.

RP using the same dataset collected from [24]. Each algorithm is executed for 10 runs for 10, 20, and 30 generations and best are noted and compared. The proposed approach achieves the highest accuracy, which is 8.8%, 7.2%, and 10.6% more than PSO, DE, and DA, respectively.

5.6   CONCLUSION

This paper proposed an optimized CAD system for the detection and diagnosis of COVID-19 using lung CT images. The strength of this proposed work lies in deriving an optimized and automatic system that uses genetic computations for segmentation using an optimal selection of threshold, feature selection, and classification and using an optimal selection of initial weights, input features, and hidden node size. The proposed work isto be implemented using a simple wrapper-based approach. The performance of the proposed work hasbeen investigated using publicly available datasets. In the future, the proposed CAD system couldbe applied for high dimensional COVID-19 datasets and couldbe also utilized for the diagnosis of other diseases.

REFERENCES

1. Novel coronavirus (2019-nCoV) situation reports. *www.who.int.* [Online]. Available: https://www.who.int/emergencies/diseases/novel-coronavirus-2019/situation-reports.
2. Kanne, J. P. (2020). Chest CT findings in 2019 novel coronavirus (2019-nCoV) Infections from Wuhan, China: Key points for the radiologist. *Radiology*, 295, 200241.
3. Bernheim, A.et al. (2020). Chest CT findings in coronavirus disease-19 (COVID-19): Relationship to duration of infection. *Radiology*, 295, 200463.
4. Xie, X., Z.Zhong, W.Zhao, C.Zheng, F.Wang, and J.Liu. (2020). Chest CT for typical 2019-nCoV pneumonia: Relationship to negative RT-PCR testing. *Radiology*, 296, 200343.
5. Wang, L., and A.Wong. (2020). COVID-Net: A tailored deep convolutional neural network design for detection of COVID-19 cases from chest X-ray images. arXiv:2003.09871 [Electrical Engineering and Systems Science.
6. Hu, Z.et al. (2020). Clinical characteristics of 24 asymptomatic infections with COVID-19 screened among close contacts in Nanjing, China. *Sci China Life Sci*, 63(5), 706–711.
7. Bullock, J., A.Luccioni, K. H.Pham, C. S. N.Lam, and M.Luengo-Oroz. (2020). Mapping the landscape of artificial intelligence applications against COVID-19. arXiv:2003.11336 [Computer Science].
8. National health commission of the people's republic of china, diagnosis and treatment protocol for COVID-19 (trial version 7). [Online] Available: *en.nhc.gov. cn/2020-03/29/c_78469.*
9. Dong, D.et al. (2020). The role of imaging in the detection and management of COVID-19: A review. *IEEE Reviews in Biomedical Engineering*, Vol: early access, Page range: 1-1
10. Shi, F.et al. (2020). Review of artificial intelligence techniques in imaging data acquisition, segmentation and diagnosis for COVID-19. *IEEE Reviews in Biomedical Engineering*, Vol: early access, Page range: 1-1
11. Ye, H.et al. (2019). Precise diagnosis of intracranial hemorrhage and subtypes using a three-dimensional joint convolutional and recurrent neural network. *European Radiology*, 29(11), 6191–6201.
12. Rajaraman, S., S.Candemir, I.Kim, G.Thoma, and S.Antani. (2018). Visualization and interpretation of convolutional neural network predictions in detecting pneumonia in pediatric chest radiographs. *Applied Sciences*, 8(10), 1715.
13. Anthimopoulos, M., S.Christodoulidis, L.Ebner, A.Christe, and S.Mougiakakou. (2016). Lung pattern classification for interstitial lung diseases using a deep convolutional neural network. *IEEE Transactions on Medical Imaging*, 35(5), 1207–1216.
14. Li, L.et al. (2020). Artificial intelligence distinguishes COVID-19 from community acquired pneumonia on chest CT. *Radiology*, 296, 200905.
15. Ozturk, T., M.Talo, E. A.Yildirim, U. B.Baloglu, O.Yildirim, and U. RajendraAcharya. (2020). Automated detection of COVID-19 cases using deep neural networks with X-ray images. *Computers in Biology and Medicine*, 121, 103792.
16. Narin, A., C.Kaya, and Z.Pamuk. (2020). Automatic detection of coronavirus disease (COVID-19) using X-ray images and deep convolutional neural networks. arXiv:2003.10849 [Electrical Engineering and Systems Science].
17. Apostolopoulos, I. D., and T. A.Mpesiana. (2020). Covid-19: Automatic detection from X-ray images utilizing transfer learning with convolutional neural networks. *Physical and Engineering Sciences in Medicine*, 43(2), 635–640.
18. Gozes, O., M. Frid-Adar, H. Greenspan, P. D. Browning, H. Zhang, W. Ji, A. Bernheim, and E. Siegel. (2020). Rapid AI development cycle for the coronavirus (COVID-19) pandemic: Initial results for automated detection & patient monitoring using deep learning CT image analysis. arXiv:2003.05037 [Electrical Engineering and Systems Science].

19. Singh, D., V. Kumar, and M. Kaur. (2020). Classification of COVID-19 patients from chest CT images using multi-objective differential evolution–based convolutional neural networks. *European Journal of Clinical Microbiology & Infectious Diseases*, 39, 1379–1389.

20. Shan, F., Y. Gao, J. Wang, W. Shi, N. Shi, M. Han, Z. Xue, D. Shen, and Y. Shi. (2020). Lung infection quantification of COVID-19 in CT images with deep learning. arXiv:2003.04655 [Computer Science].

21. Xu, X., X. Jiang, C. Ma, P. Du, X. Li, S. Lv, L. Yu, Y. Chen, J. Su, G. Lang, Y. Li, H. Zhao, K. Xu, L. Ruan, and W. Wu. (2020). Deep learning system to screen coronavirus disease 2019 pneumonia. arXiv:2002.09334 [Physics].

22. Wang, S., B. Kang, J. Ma, X. Zeng, M. Xiao, J. Guo, M. Cai, J. Yang, Y. Li, X. Meng, and B. Xu. (2020). A deep learning algorithm using CT images to screen for corona virus disease (COVID-19). MedRxiv.

23. Sethy, P. K., and S. K.Behera. (2020). Detection of coronavirus disease (COVID-19) based on deep features. *www.preprints.org*.

24. UCSD-AI4H. (2020). UCSD-AI4H/COVID-CT. *GitHub*, 06-May-2020. [Online]. Available: https://github.com/UCSD-AI4H/COVID-CT.

6 Micro-Expression Recognition Using 3D-CNN Layering

Prerit Rathi, Rajat Sharma, Prateek Singal,
Puneet Singh Lamba, Gopal Chaudhary,
and Fadi Al-Turjman

CONTENTS

6.1   INTRODUCTION

Facial expressions best depict the emotional state and intentions of an individual. Micro-expressions are the best means to identify deception and the cognitive thinking of an individual [1]. The credible research in the study of facial expressions is attributed to Ekman and Friesen [2]. Ekman's research has been attributed to being the foundation of many studies in the psychology of emotions. They characterized seven main types of emotions: happy, sad, anger, surprise, fear, contempt, and disgust, and these were considered as comprehensive emotions [3, 4]. However, recent studies argue that these emotions are regional and culturally determined, rather than being universal [5]. Micro-expressions include notable amounts of information regarding the actual emotions, which can be useful in pragmatic applications such as intelligence, security, and interrogations.

Facial expressions can be static or dynamic [6]. Static only extracts information from single spatial frames, whereas dynamic provides a cognitive result using temporal sequencing of continuous frames [7]. Traditional methods used shallow learning [8] (such as "Local Binary Pattern" and "Matrix factorization"). Recently, deep learning methods, like CNN (Convolutional Neural Network) [9,10], have provided more credibility and accuracy in the study of micro-expressions and other computer vision problems.

Despite the computational supremacy of CNN, some challenges posed by FER are:

  (i) Significantly huge training data required to avoid overfitting.
  (ii) Different personal attributes give inter-subject variations [11].

Additionally, variations in pose and illumination are also common. Thus, deep networks that cater to large intra-class variations are required.

Going further, the paper can be organized as: literature review of the existing technologies; existing data set comparison; comprehensive methodology of the proposed solution; and lastly, the experimental results and analysis.

6.2   LITERATURE REVIEW

The literature review can be classified into two sections – the older hand-designed (manual) methods and the current learning-based (dynamic) methods.

6.2.1   HAND-DESIGNED (MANUAL) TECHNIQUES

Some of the prominent works were by: Wu – the "Support Vector Machine (SVM)" [12] used over the characteristics produced to identify facial expressions. Polikovsky utilized the descriptor of the 3D gradient-oriented histogram for finding the association among the frames by dividing the face into several sub-regions [13,14], and Pfister used the descriptors for local Spatio-temporal [15] texture to understand micro-expressions. Most of the other works, including those by Liu, Zhao, Huang [16,17], were also based on SVM for facial expression recognition.

6.2.2   Learning-Based (Dynamic) Techniques

Advances in computing techniques based on GPU allows for the training of large datasets. Learning-based methods like classification, detection, and segmentation [18] can be applied to computer vision problems. Convolutional Neural Network (CNN) is the current trend for using deep machine learning in Computer-Vision R&D [19]. Techniques like augmentation to generate synthetic images and to train Deep CNN were used by Takalkar et al. [20]. This, in turn, generates the features of optical flow, which are inputted to the SVM for it to train and recognize them. The interpolated image output is fed into a DCNN to classify the expressions [21, 22]. The main disadvantage of using this technique is the loss of temporal data. Fine tuning in the form of pre-trained CNN of imageNet and 3D CNN have been used by Peng and Li respectively [23, 24], among others. Many other models, such as those by Hasani and Satya, have made efforts to classify micro-expressions into two-step architecture. Firstly, spatial features from each frame are extracted using a CNN-based model, and this is inputted into random fields that are continuous and linearly linked to determine the temporal correlation amongst the selected frames. Duan uses LTOP [25, 26, 27] to recognize eye regions over the above two steps. Sai Prasanna Teja Reddy et al. have made efforts in analyzing the importance and role of prominent facial features, apart from the eyes and mouth region, in extracting the micro-expressions using the MicroExpSTCNN and MicroExpFuseNet models based on 3D Convolutional Neural Networks [28]. Thus, the main advantage of Deep Learning-based dynamic algorithms over Hand-designed features is that they are more robust and have better accuracy and performance [29]. Even now, the usage of 3D-CNN-based models for micro-expression recognition is restricted, and additional knowledge like optical-flow, etc. [29] is used.

6.3   MICRO-EXPRESSIONS DATASETS

6.3.1   Non-Spontaneous Dataset

The earliest datasets were non-spontaneous datasets, which were mainly of three types.

6.3.1.1   Polikovsky Dataset

Table 6.1 summarizes the Polikovsky dataset. The major drawbacks of this dataset were its limited access and the fact that posed expressions are not representative of spontaneous human expressions [30].

TABLE 6.1
Polikovsky Dataset

Frame Speed	Resolution	Sample Size
200fps	640×480	70 Posed Expressions

6.3.1.2 USF-HD

This dataset (as summarized in Table 6.2) is not available for public use, and the low frame capture speed may result in a loss of critical information. Moreover, only four emotions were captured instead of the universal seven [31].

6.3.1.3 York DDT

Two types of clips, emotional (stressful) and non-emotional (neutral), were classified [31]. Inaccessibility to the public domain and the low frame rate are the major issues with this dataset. Table 6.3 shows the snapshot of the dataset.

6.3.2 SPONTANEOUS DATASETS

Since micro-expressions are difficult to fake, it is very difficult to make a spontaneous dataset large enough to carry out error-free research, and thus, the main challenge was to bring out the true emotions and expressions. Some of the spontaneous datasets are:

6.3.2.1 CASME

Chinese Academy of Sciences Micro-expressions, better known as CASME, as explained in Table 6.4, was created by Yan et al. For Class A, natural lighting was used whereas two light-emitting-diodes lights were availed for Class B.

TABLE 6.2
USF-HD Dataset

Frame Speed	Sample Size
29.7fps	100 Posed Expressions

TABLE 6.3
York DDT Dataset

Frame Speed	Resolution	Sample Size
25fps	320×240	20 video clips

TABLE 6.4
CASME Dataset

Frame Speed	Resolution		Sample Size
	Class A	Class B	
60fps	1280×720	640×480	195

6.3.2.2 SMIC

Spontaneous micro-expressions corpus was created by Li et al. [32]. The dataset is the spontaneous reaction of 20 participants to a specific movie clip. Three types of datasets were used: HS (high-speed camera) [33], VIS (basic visual camera) [34] and NIR (near-infrared) as shown in Table 6.5. Figure 6.1 shows a sample of HS SMIC dataset with negative expressions.

6.3.2.3 CASME II

CASME II is a mixture of all spontaneous and dynamic images saved as MJPEG format [35], which were labeled as action units (AU) and based on facial action coding (FACS). Table 6.6 gives a brief summary of the dataset, and a sample of faces with the happiness emotion is shown in Figure 6.2.

6.3.2.4 SAMM Dataset

Spontaneous actions and micro-movements, better known as SAMM (as summarized in Table 6.7), was the first high-resolution dataset with large spontaneous variability of demographics, and was tailored explicitly for each individual, depicting all the seven basic universal emotions [35]. Figure 6.3 shows a sample expression.

6.3.2.5 CAS(ME)^2

CAS(ME)^2 is a dataset of spontaneous macro- and micro-expressions, developed by Qu et al. [36] (as expounded in Table 6.8) at CAS using 22 participants with a mean age of 22.59 years. It comprised of 250 macro- and 53 micro-expressions that depicted four basic emotions [37].

TABLE 6.5
SMIC Dataset

Data Set	Frame Speed	Resolution	Positive	Negative	Surprised	Total
HS	100fps	640×480	51	70	43	164
VIS	25	640×480	28	23	20	71
NIR	25	640×480	28	23	20	71

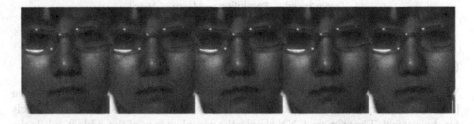

FIGURE 6.1   Sample of HS SMIC dataset with negative expressions.

TABLE 6.6
CASME II Dataset

Frame Size	Resolution	Sample Size
200fps	640×480	247

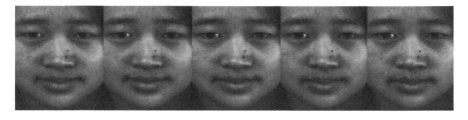

FIGURE 6.2   CASME II dataset with happiness expression.

TABLE 6.7
SAMM Dataset

Frame Speed	Resolution	Sample Size
200fps	2040×1088	159

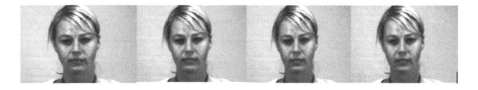

FIGURE 6.3   SAMM dataset with anger expression.

TABLE 6.8
CAS(ME)² Dataset

		Sample Size	
Frame Speed	**Resolution**	**Macro**	**Micro**
30fps	640×480	250	53

6.4   PROPOSED CNN MODELS

We all know CNN models are better able to map spatial and temporal information [38] in micro-expression recognition; that is why we selected two 3D CNN models for this project. The primary CNN checks the complete face of the subject, while the secondary CNN focuses solely on the eyes and mouth.

6.4.1 PRIMARY CNN

The Primary 3D-CNN will focus on the complete face of the subject. The architecture is shown in Figure 6.4. The input dimension for Primary CNN is width × height × depth, where width and height are affixed to 64 in the experimental setup, and the depth value is based upon the available set of data [39]. This CNN would consist of layers for 3D conv, 3D Maxpool, fully interconnected layers, correlated activation functions, and finally, dropout layer.

As the convolution layer is 3-dimensional, it is able to extract both spatial and temporal information. As for the Maxpool segment, it is used to decrease the output dimensions received from the conv layer, keeping the principal features intact [40]. The 3D Maxpool layer chooses the most prominent features in a short space and time frame. Finally, dropout helps reduce overfitting by adding regularization for the system [41]. The flat layer just stretches multidimensional values into a 1D array for the next layer. A fully connected layer (aka denser layer) provides non-linearity into the system. In the end, the SoftMax layer produces a class score for all the classes of the dataset. Our proposed system comprises stacking one 3-dimensional conv layer with utmost 32 filters of dimensions $3 \times 3 \times 15$, one 3D Maxpool layer with kernel size $3 \times 3 \times 3$, and two fully connected layers (dense layer).

The end dimensions of the denser layer rely upon the number of all the labeled expressions present in our dataset. Table 6.9 displays dimensions of the layers used. The output dimension varies as per the dataset being used.

6.4.2 SECONDARY CNN

While the function of the primary CNN considered the whole face area, the secondary CNN emphasizes the eyes and mouth, as they are more instrumental in expression analysis [42]. Consequently, we propose the secondary CNN be focused on the

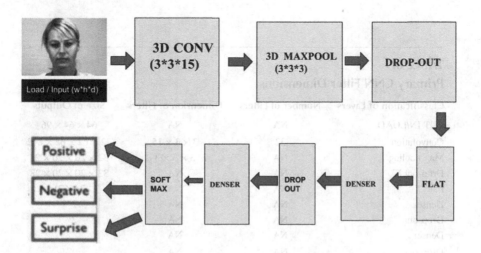

FIGURE 6.4 Primary CNN architecture.

eyes and mouth area as input into two distinct 3D CNNs, both of which are fused later on. For this task, we propose the use of DLib face detector, which uses 68 landmarks [42] in the face to detect a face. Further, we suggest two variations for the secondary CNN: intermediate fusion or late fusion.

Intermediate Fusion: The characteristic features of both the 3-dimensional Convolutional Neural Networks (eye CNN and mouth CNN) are fused at some midpoint [43, 44]. The suggested layer-architecture is presented in Figure 6.5. The suggested secondary model has two distinct 3-fimensional Convolutional Neural Networks, with both the networks built by stacking, one 3-dimensional convolutional layer with 32 filters of dimensions $3 \times 3 \times 15$, and one 3-dimensional Maxpool layer with the dimensions of kernel $3 \times 3 \times 3$. The flatten layer converts activation map into a 1D vector [45]. The flattened features are then concatenated to get a different vector. With this fusion, the features are consecutively changed and processed with dense and dropout just before the final class score is generated. Table 6.10 provides further details.

Late Fusion: here, the features are merged right before the last denser layer. Both eyes and mouth are fed to distinct CNNs and then merged amongst themselves at the final, completely connected layer (dense layer). The suggested model architecture is displayed in Figure 6.6. The pair of distinct Convolutional Neural Network consists of stacks, one 3-dimensional convolutional layer having 32 filters with dimensions $3 \times 3 \times 15$, one 3-dimensional Maxpool layer with the kernel dimensions of $3 \times 3 \times 3$, and the flat layer to attain a singular dimensional vector [46, 47]. The dropout, flat and denser layers are utilized in both the systems [48, 49]. The pair of networks are merged before the last denser layer. Table 6.11 displays the system design of the late fusion, filter sizes, and final dimensions of various used layers.

TABLE 6.9
Primary CNN Filter Dimensions

Classification of Layers	Number of Filters	Dimension of Filters	Size of Outputs
PUT IN/LOAD	NA	NA	$64 \times 64 \times 96$
Convolution	32	$3 \times 3 \times 15$	$32 \times 62 \times 62 \times 842$
Max Pooling	NA	$3 \times 3 \times 3$	$32 \times 20 \times 20 \times 28$
Drop-out	NA	NA	$32 \times 20 \times 20 \times 28$
Flat	NA	NA	345621
Denser	NA	NA	2^7
Drop-out	NA	NA	2^7
Denser	NA	NA	2
Drop-out	NA	NA	2

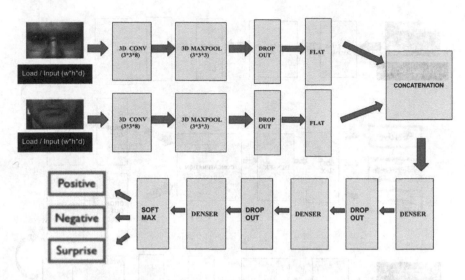

FIGURE 6.5 Secondary CNN (intermediate) architecture.

TABLE 6.10

Secondary CNN Filter Dimensions (Intermediate)

Classification of Layers	Dimension of Filters	Size of Outputs
Load-1	NA	$30 \times 32 \times 96$
Load-2	NA	$30 \times 32 \times 96$
3D-Convolution-1	$3 \times 3 \times 15$	$32 \times 30 \times 30 \times 82$
3D-Convolution-2	$3 \times 3 \times 15$	$32 \times 30 \times 30 \times 82$
3D-Maxpooling-1	$3 \times 3 \times 3$	$32 \times 10 \times 10 \times 27$
3D-Maxpooling-2	$3 \times 3 \times 3$	$32 \times 10 \times 10 \times 27$
Drop-out – 1	NA	$32 \times 20 \times 20 \times 27$
Drop-out – 2	NA	$32 \times 20 \times 20 \times 27$
Flat(1)	NA	86420
Flat(2)	NA	86420
Concatenation	NA	86420
Denser	NA	2^{10}
Drop-out	NA	2^{10}
Denser	NA	2^{7}
Drop-out	NA	2^{7}
Denser	NA	2

6.5 EXPERIMENTAL RESULTS AND DISCUSSIONS

The result of this model in the environment, along with its stability and effect on variance, is compared with other models [50, 51] along with the 3D kernel size.

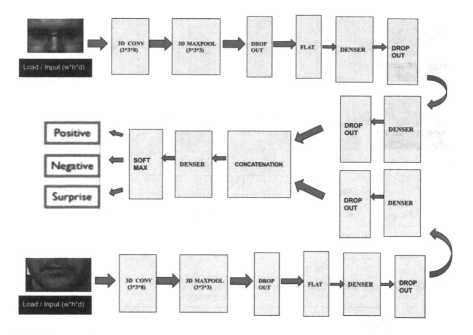

FIGURE 6.6   Secondary CNN (late) architecture.

Figure 6.7 depicts the accuracy comparison of the existing methods (in blue) with the accuracy of the proposed models (in orange) over the SMIC dataset.

6.5.1   EXPERIMENTAL RESULTS

The results for the suggested primary and secondary CNN models with hand-made methods (HCM) and deep learning dynamic methods (DLM) are shown in Table 6.12, using the SMIC dataset. The accuracy of other cited methods has been taken from their respective source papers [54]. The primary CNN that is proposed performs better than other cited methods over the dataset of SMIC. The performance of the suggested secondary CNN (chiefly intermediate fusion) is an improvement over current method. Using joint training in space and time with 3-dimensional Convolutional Neural Network in both the proposed CNNs allows for more precise extraction of information for micro-expression recognition purposes. Among both proposed CNNs, the primary CNN model is better than the secondary model. The late fusion secondary CNN performs better for the SMIC dataset.

6.5.2   ACCURACY STANDARD DEVIATION ANALYSIS

In the results, we recorded the standard deviation along with accuracy to highlight the model's stability and for fewer training data [55]. Table 6.13 displays the standard deviation and mean validation accuracies for primary CNN and secondary CNN for both datasets from epochs 91 to 100. It is observed that the suggested CNNs exhibit good stability over SMIC datasets, while CAS(ME)^2 is rational.

TABLE 6.11
Secondary CNN Filter Dimensions (Late)

Classification of Layers	Dimension of Filters	Size of Outputs
Load-1	NA	$30 \times 32 \times 96$
Load-2	NA	$30 \times 32 \times 96$
3D-Convolution - 1	$3 \times 3 \times 15$	$32 \times 30 \times 30 \times 82$
3D-Convolution - 2	$3 \times 3 \times 15$	$32 \times 30 \times 30 \times 82$
3D-Maxpool-1	$3 \times 3 \times 3$	$32 \times 10 \times 10 \times 27$
3D-Maxpool-2	$3 \times 3 \times 3$	$32 \times 10 \times 10 \times 27$
Drop-out-1	NA	$32 \times 10 \times 10 \times 27$
Drop-out-2	NA	$32 \times 10 \times 10 \times 27$
Flat-1	NA	86420
Flat-2	NA	86420
Denser-1	NA	2^10
Drop-out-1	NA	2^10
Denser-2	NA	2^10
Drop-out-2	NA	2^10
Denser-3	NA	2^7
Drop-out-3	NA	2^7
Denser-4	NA	2^7
Drop-out-3	NA	2^7
Concatenation	NA	2^8
Denser	NA	2

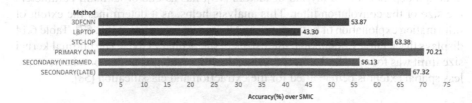

FIGURE 6.7   Accuracy comparison.

TABLE 6.12
Results and Comparison

Method	Published	Type	Dataset-SMIC
LBPTOP[50]	Year-2013	Hand Crafted Methods	43.30%
STC-LQP[51]	Year-2016	Hand Crafted Methods	63.38%
Augmented CNN[52]	Year-2017	Deep Learning Methods	NA
3DFCNN[53]	Year-2018	Deep Learning Methods	53.87%
Primary CNN	Proposed	Deep Learning Methods	70.21%
Secondary CNN (intermediate fusion)	Proposed	Deep Learning Methods	56.13%
Secondary CNN (late fusion)	Proposed	Deep Learning Methods	67.32%

TABLE 6.13
Standard Deviation

| Dataset | Primary CNN | Secondary CNN | |
		Intermediate Fusion	Late Fusion
SMIC	$63.05 \pm 2.48\%$	$50.02 \pm 4.65\%$	$60.59 \pm 3.91\%$

TABLE 6.14
Accuracy of Different Filters

Filter Size	Accuracy (%)	Filter Size	Accuracy (%)
$3 \times 3 \times 3$	82.39	$5 \times 5 \times 15$	51.22
$3 \times 3 \times 7$	80.94	$5 \times 5 \times 19$	29.72
$3 \times 3 \times 15$	87.80	$7 \times 7 \times 3$	70.37
$3 \times 3 \times 19$	29.72	$7 \times 7 \times 7$	51.22
$5 \times 5 \times 3$	63.03	$7 \times 7 \times 15$	29.72
$5 \times 5 \times 7$	58.45	$7 \times 7 \times 19$	51.22

6.5.3 EFFECT OF 3D KERNEL

The principle behind the design of the model is 3D convolution. Performance, although dependent on a myriad of factors [15], has as one of its main parameters the size of the convolution filter. This analysis helps, as it determines the extent of information exploitation of both spatial and temporal information [56, 57]. Table 6.14 displays the accuracy of multiple filter sizes in the primary CNN. The optimal kernel size limit was found to be $3 \times 3 \times 15$. Also, the filter with greater temporal extent and less spatial extent is better suited for the extraction and classification [58].

6.5.4 IMPACT OF FACIAL FEATURES

Here, we try to explain the reason for our primary CNNs enhanced performance over both our late and intermediate secondary CNN versions. It's obvious that model success depends on the prominent features it grasps during training cycles [59]. We developed models presuming that both eyes and mouth provide more to the micro-expressions. Thus, we examined saliency maps to find out significant facial features. It helps to calculate the positive response towards the generation of the final class score [59]. The saliency maps are given in Figure 6.8, presented with the earliest seven frames for four unique videos at different times. It is observed that other facial features prove necessary to identify the micro-expressions apart from the eyes and mouth [60, 61]. This may probably be one of the reasons behind the success that our primary CNN appears to produce better than the secondary CNN [62].

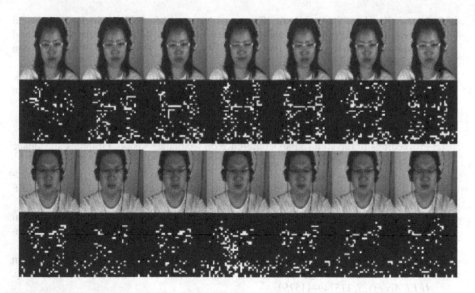

FIGURE 6.8   Saliency map to understand facial features.

6.6   CONCLUSION

This paper analyzes the existing techniques and suggests two Convolutional Neural Networks in three dimensions (two spatial and one temporal) for recognizing the micro expressions from images. The 3D-CNN technique is utilized to enter convolution (both spatial and temporal), which leads to training of dataset spatio-temporally at the same time. Our intensive studies on the two suggested CNN models over the standard dataset SMIC reveals that other important facial regions may also contribute in recognizing micro expressions, and not just eyes and mouth regions alone. We have found the reliability of our system over the SMIC database, which is considered amongst the best of the known databases. The effect kernel size is also analyzed, resulting in smaller spatial and finer dimensional filters.

REFERENCES

1. Ekman, P. (2009). Lie catching and Micro Expressions. In Martin, C. (Ed.), The Philosophy of Deception (Vol. 1, p. 5), New York, NY: Oxford University Press.
2. Takalkar, M., M. Xu, Q. Wu, and Z. Chaczko. (2018). A survey: Facial micro-expression recognition. In *Multimedia Tools and Applications*, 77(15), 19301–19325.
3. Li, Xiaobai, Xiaopeng Hong, Antti Moilanen, Xiaohua Huang, Tomas Pfister, Guoying Zhao, and Matti Pietikäinen. (2017). Towards reading hidden emotions: A comparative study of spontaneous micro-expression spotting and recognition methods. *IEEE Transactions on Affective Computing*, 9(4), 563–577.
4. Merghani, W., A. K. Davison, and M. H. Yap. (2018). A review on facial micro-expressions analysis: datasets, features and metrics. arXiv:1805.02397.

5. Huang, Xiaohua, Su-Jing Wang, Guoying Zhao, and Matti Piteikainen. 2015. Facial micro-expression recognition using spatiotemporal local binary pattern with integral projection. In Proceedings of the IEEE international conference on computer vision workshops (pp. 1–9).
6. Wang, Y., J. See, R. C-W. Phan, and Y.-H. Oh. (2014). Lbp with six intersection points: Reducing redundant information in lbp-top for micro-expression recognition. In Asian Conference on Computer Vision (pp. 525–537). Springer.
7. Mukherjee, S., B. Vamshi, K. V. S. V. K. Rcddy, R. V. Krishna, and S. V. S. Harish. (2016). Recognizing facial expressions using novel motion based features. In Proceedings of the 10th Indian Conference on Computer Vision, Graphics and Image Processing (pp. 1–8).
8. Liu, Y.-J., J.-K. Zhang, W.-J. Yan, S.-J. Wang, G. Zhao, and X. Fu. (2015). A main directional mean optical flow feature for spontaneous micro-expression recognition. *IEEE Transactions on Affective Computing*, 7(4), 299–310.
9. Jacob, S., V. G. Menon, F. Al-Turjman, P. G. Vinoj, and L. Mostarda. (2019). Artificial muscle intelligence system with deep learning for post-stroke assistance and rehabilitation. *IEEE Access*, 7, 133463–133473.
10. Al-Turjman, F, H. Zahmatkesh, and L. Mostarda. (2019). Quantifying uncertainty in internet of medical things and big-data services using intelligence and deep learning. *IEEE Access*, 7, 115749–115759.
11. Chen, L.-C., G. Papandreou, I. Kokkinos, K. Murphy, and A. L. Yuille. (2017). Deeplab: Semantic image segmentation with deep convolutional nets, atrous convolution, and fully connected crfs. *IEEE Transactions on Pattern Analysis and Machine Intelligence*, 40(4), 834–848.
12. Hou, W., X. Gao, D. Tao, and X. Li. (2014). Blind image quality assessment via deep learning. *IEEE Transactions on Neural Networks and Learning Systems*, 26(6), 1275–1286.
13. Nagpal, C., and S. R. Dubey. (2019). A performance evaluation of convolutional neu ral networks for face anti spoofing. In 2019 International Joint Conference on Neural Networks (IJCNN) (pp. 1–8). IEEE.
14. Basha, S. H. S., S. Ghosh, K. K. Babu, S. R. Dubey, V. Pulabaigari, and S. Mukherjee. (2018). Rccnet: An efficient convolutional neural network for histological routine colon cancer nuclei classification. In 2018 15th International Conference on Control, Automation, Robotics and Vision (ICARCV) (pp. 1222–1227). IEEE.
15. Hasani, B., and M. H. Mahoor. (2017). Spatio-temporal facial expression recognition using convolutional neural networks and conditional random fields. In 2017 12th IEEE International Conference on Automatic Face & Gesture Recognition (FG 2017) (pp. 790–795). IEEE.
16. Guo, J., S. Zhou, J. Wu, J. Wan, X. Zhu, Z. Lei, and S. Z. Li. (2017). Multi-modality network with visual and geometrical information for micro emotion recognition. In 2017 12th IEEE International Conference on Automatic Face & Gesture Recognition (FG 2017) (pp. 814–819). IEEE.
17. Gan, Y. S., S.-T. Liong, W.-C. Yau, Y.-C. Huang, and L.-K. Tan. (2019). Off-apexnet on micro-expression recognition system. *Signal Processing: Image Communication*, 74, 129–139.
18. V. Satya. (2018). *Revealing True Emotions Through Micro-Expressions: A Machine Learning Approach*. CMU SEI Insights.
19. Patel, D., X. Hong, and G. Zhao. (2016). Selective deep features for micro-expression recognition. In 2016 23rd International Conference on Pattern Recognition (ICPR) (pp. 2258–2263). IEEE.

20. Takalkar, M., and M. Xu. (2017). Image based facial micro-expression recognition using deep learning on small datasets. *International Conference on Digital Image Computing: Techniques and Applications (DICTA)*.
21. Polikovsky, S., Y. Kameda, and Y. Ohta. (2009). Facial micro-expressions recognition using high speed camera and 3D-gradient descriptor. In 3rd International Conference on Imaging for Crime Detection and Prevention (ICDP 2009) (p. 16). IEEE.
22. Lu, H., K. Kpalma, and J. Ronsin. (2018). Motion descriptors for micro-expression recognition. *Signal Processing: Image Communication*, 67 , 108–117.
23. Shreve, M., S. Godavarthy, D. Goldgof, and S. Sarkar. (2011). Macro-and micro-expression spotting in long videos using spatio-temporal strain. In *Face and Gesture* (pp. 51–56). IEEE.
24. Pfister, T., X. Li, G. Zhao, and M. Pietikäinen. (2011). Recognising spontaneous facial micro-expressions. In 2011 International Conference on Computer Vision (pp. 1449–1456). IEEE.
25. Zhao, G., and M. Pietikainen. (2007). Dynamic texture recognition using local binary patterns with an application to facial expressions. *IEEE Transactions on Pattern Analysis and Machine Intelligence*, 29(6), 915–928.
26. Wang, Y., H. Yu, B. Stevens, and H. Liu. (2015). Dynamic facial expression recognition using local patch and lbp-top. In 2015 8th International Conference on Human System Interaction (HSI) (pp. 362–367). IEEE
27. Duan, X., Q. Dai, X. Wang, Y. Wang, and Z. Hua. Recognizing spontaneous micro-expression from eye region. *Neurocomputing*, 217, 27–36.
28. Reddy, S. P. T., S. T. Karri, S. R. Dubey, and S. Mukherjee. (2019). Spontaneous facial micro-expression recognition using 3D spatiotemporal convolutional neural networks. In 2019 International Joint Conference on Neural Networks (IJCNN) (pp. 1–8). IEEE.
29. Grobova, J., M. Colovic, M. Marjanovic, A. Njegus, H. Demire, and G. Anbarjafari. (2017). Automatic hidden sadness detection using micro-expressions. In 2017 12th IEEE International Conference on Automatic Face & Gesture Recognition (FG 2017) (pp. 828–832). IEEE.
30. Li, X., J. Yu, and S. Zhan. (2016). Spontaneous facial micro-expression detection based on deep learning. In 2016 IEEE 13th International Conference on Signal Processing (ICSP) (pp. 1130–1134). IEEE.
31. Li, Q., J. Yu, T. Kurihara, and S. Zhan. (2018). Micro-expression analysis by fusing deep convolutional neural network and optical flow. In 2018 5th International Conference on Control, Decision and Information Technologies (CoDIT) (pp. 265–270). IEEE.
32. Mayya, V., R. M. Pai, and M. M. M. Pai. Combining temporal interpolation and DCNN for faster recognition of micro-expressions in video sequences. In 2016 International Conference on Advances in Computing, Communications and Informatics (ICACCI) (pp. 699–703). IEEE.
33. Wang, S.-J., B.-J. Li, Y.-J. Liu, W.-J. Yan, X. Ou, X. Huang, F. Xu, and X. Fu. (2018). Micro-expression recognition with small sample size by transferring long-term convolutional neural network. *Neurocomputing*, 312, 251–262.
34. Peng, M., Z. Wu, Z. Zhang, and T. Chen. (20128). From macro to micro expression recognition: Deep learning on small datasets using transfer learning. In 2018 13th IEEE International Conference on Automatic Face & Gesture Recognition (FG 2018) (pp. 657–661). IEEE.
35. Kim, D. H., W. J. Baddar, and Y. M. Ro. (2016). Micro-expression recognition with expression-state constrained spatio-temporal feature representations. In Proceedings of the 24th ACM international conference on Multimedia (pp. 382–386). AC Med
36. Kim, D. H., W. J. Baddar, J. Jang, and Y. M. Ro. Multi-objective based spatio-temporal feature representation learning robust to expression intensity variations for facial expression recognition. *IEEE Transactions on Affective Computing*, 10(2), 223–236.

37. Khor, H.-Q., J. See, R. C. W. Phan, and W. Lin. (2018). Enriched long-term recurrent convolutional network for facial micro-expression recognition. In 2018 13th IEEE International Conference on Automatic Face & Gesture Recognition (FG 2018) (pp. 667–674). IEEE.

38. Peng, M., C. Wang, T. Chen, G. Liu, and X. Fu. (2017). Dual temporal scale convolutional neural network for micro-expression recognition. *Frontiers in Psychology*, 8, 1745.

39. Srivastava, N., G. Hinton, A. Krizhevsky, I. Sutskever, and R. Salakhutdinov. (2014). Dropout: A simple way to prevent neural networks from overfitting. *Journal of Machine Learning Research*, 15(1), 1929–1958.

40. Iwasaki, M., and Y. Noguchi. (2016). Hiding true emotions: Micro-expressions in eyes retrospectively concealed by mouth movements. *Scientific Reports*, 6, 22049.

41. Agrawal, D. D., S. R. Dubey, and A. S. Jalal. Emotion recognition from facial expressions based on multi-level classification. *International Journal of Computational Vision and Robotics*, 4(4), 365–389.

42. Qu, F., S.-J. Wang, W.-J. Yan, H. Li, S. Wu, and X. Fu. (2017). CAS (ME) $^$ 2$: A database for spontaneous macro-expression and micro-expression spotting and recognition. *IEEE Transactions on Affective Computing*, 9(4), 424–436.

43. Mollahosseini, A., B. Hasani, and M. H. Mahoor. (2017). Affectnet: A database for facial expression, valence, and arousal computing in the wild. *IEEE Transactions on Affective Computing*, 10(1), 18–31.

44. Zhang, Z., P. Luo, C. C. Loy, and X. Tang. (2018). From facial expression recognition to interpersonal relation prediction. *International Journal of Computer Vision*, 126(5), 550–569.

45. Dhall, A., R. Goecke, S. Lucey, and T. Gedeon. (2012). Collecting large, richly annotated facial-expression databases from movies. *IEEE Multimedia*, 3, 34–41.

46. Dhall, A., R. Goecke, S. Lucey, and T. Gedeon. (2011). Acted facial expressions in the wild database. In *Australian National University, Canberra, Australia,* Technical Report TR-CS-11, 2, 1.

47. Dhall, A., R. Goecke, S. Lucey, and T. Gedeon. (2011). Static facial expression analysis in tough conditions: Data, evaluation protocol and benchmark. In 2011 IEEE International Conference on Computer Vision Workshops (ICCV Workshops) (pp. 2106–2112). IEEE.

48. Benitez-Quiroz, C. F., R. Srinivasan, Q. Feng, Y. Wang, and A. M. Martinez. (2017). Emotionet challenge: Recognition of facial expressions of emotion in the wild. arXiv:1703.01210.

49. Du, S., Y. Tao, and A. M. Martinez. Compound facial expressions of emotion. *Proceedings of the National Academy of Sciences of the United States of America*, 111(15), E1454–E1462.

50. Li, X., T. Pfister, X. Huang, G. Zhao, and M. Pietikäinen. (2013). A spontaneous micro-expression database: Inducement, collection and baseline. In 2013 10th IEEE International Conference and Workshops on Automatic Face and Gesture Recognition (FG) (pp. 1–6). IEEE.

51. Huang, X., G. Zhao, X. Hong, W. Zheng, and M. Pietikäinen. (2016). Spontaneous facial micro-expression analysis using spatiotemporal completed local quantized patterns. *Neurocomputing* (Volume 175, Part A), 175, 564–578.

52. Takalkar, M. A., and M. Xu. Image based facial micro-expression recognition using deep learning on small datasets. In 2017 International Conference on Digital Image Computing: Techniques and Applications (DICTA) (pp. 1–7). IEEE.

53. Li, J., Y. Wang, J. See, and W. Liu. (2019). Micro-expression recognition based on 3D flow convolutional neural network. *Pattern Analysis and Applications*, 22(4), 1331–1339.

54. Cootes, T. F., G. J. Edwards, and C. J. Taylor. (201). Active appearance models. *IEEE Transactions on Pattern Analysis and Machine Intelligence*, 23(6), 681–685.

55. Zeng, N., H. Zhang, B. Song, W. Liu, Y. Li, and A. M. Dobaie. (2018). Facial expression recognition via learning deep sparse autoencoders. *Neurocomputing*, 273, 643–649.

56. Zhu, X., and D. Ramanan. (2012). Face detection, pose estimation, and landmark localization in the wild. In 2012 IEEE Conference on Computer Vision and Pattern Recognition (pp. 2879–2886). IEEE.

57. Kahou, S. E., C. Pal, X. Bouthillier, P. Froumenty, Ç. Gülçehre, R. Memisevic, P. Vincent et al. (2013). Combining modality specific deep neural networks for emotion recognition in video. In Proceedings of the 15th ACM on International Conference on Multimodal Interaction (pp. 543–550). AC Med

58. Devries, T., K. Biswaranjan, and G. W. Taylor. (2014). Multi-task learning of facial landmarks and expression. In 2014 Canadian Conference on Computer and Robot Vision (pp. 98–103). IEEE.

59. Asthana, A., S. Zafeiriou, S. Cheng, and M. Pantic. (2013). Robust discriminative response map fitting with constrained local models. In Proceedings of the IEEE Conference on Computer Vision and Pattern Recognition (pp. 3444–3451). IEEE.

60. Shin, M., M. Kim, and D.-S. Kwon. (2016). Baseline CNN structure analysis for facial expression recognition. In 2016 25th IEEE International Symposium on Robot and Human Interactive Communication (RO-MAN) (pp. 724–729). IEEE.

61. Meng, Z., P. Liu, J. Cai, S. Han, and Y. Tong. (2017). Identity-aware convolutional neural network for facial expression recognition. In 2017 12th IEEE International Conference on Automatic Face & Gesture Recognition (FG 2017) (pp. 558–565). IEEE.

62. Xiong, X., and F. De la Torre. (2013). Supervised descent method and its applications to face alignment. In Proceedings of the IEEE Conference on Computer Vision and Pattern Recognition (pp. 532–539). IEEE.

7 Applications of AI, IoT, IoMT, and Biosensing Devices in Curbing COVID-19

Basil Bartholomew Duwa, Mehmet Ozsoz, and Fadi Al-Turjman

CONTENTS

7.1 INTRODUCTION

Corona viruses are contagious viruses that belong to single-strand RNA viruses (corona viridae). The World Health Organization (WHO) termed coronaviruses as a global health threat. Coronaviruses are designed as round-shaped positive single-stranded viruses sized form about 600A degree–1400A degree in diameter. Coronavirus was etymologically derived from a Latin word "Corona" which means "crown." It was named by two scientists (David Tyrell and June Almeida) in 1968.

The coronaviruses are roughly spherical, large particles with spikes. The diameter of the virus is 125 nm. The part of the corona virus, diameter, and envelope is about 85 nm, and the spikes are about 20 nm [3].

The bizarre evolution of the SARS-CoV emanated in the Guandong religion of the people's Republic of China and subsequently spread to about 37 global states, leading to more than 8000 individuals infected and more than 774 deaths. Meanwhile, the pioneer hit of the MERS-CoV was recorded in Saudi Arabia, which subsequently spread to all the Middle Eastern states, which recorded about 871 deaths. The viral COVID-19 outbreak was recorded on the 31 December 2019 with a history of individuals with pneumonia. This virus is characterized by its severe contagious traits and an incubation period of 14 days. It was observed that an individual can be infected through contact with an infected person unknowingly, which leads to a high number of infections. Researchers have shown that SARS-CoV could be eliminated by a casual exposure to heat and also ultraviolet light (UV) [4] (Table 7.1).

7.1.1 CLINICAL PROPERTIES

The coronavirus 2019 can be characterized into three (3) clinical properties, multi organ dysfunction syndrome (MODS), asymptomatic state, and acute respiratory distress syndrome (ARDS). The COVID-19 cases were examined to have exhibited different clinical features, such as pneumonia cold, anorexia, dyspnea, headache, nausea, diarrhea, and so on. The United Centers for Disease Control and Prevention (CDC) says individuals above age of 60 and those having existing illness such as hypertension, asthma, heart diseases, and diabetes are at high risk of getting infected (Table 7.2).

TABLE 7.1
Places Affected by COVID-19 and Mortality Rate

Place (Country)	Mortality
USA	1,003,974
Spain	212,297
Italy	203,591
UK	165,225
Germany	159,119
France	127,060
Turkey	117,589
Russia	106,498
Iran	93,657
China	84,373

Data Source: WHO Situation Report – 30 April 2020

TABLE 7.2

Common Symptoms of COVID-19

Symptoms	Percentage (%)
Dyspnea	38.9
Fever	87.9
Anorexia	18.6
Dry cough	67.7
Myalgia	14.8
Nausea	5.0
Headache	13.6
Hemoptysis	0.9

Source: WHO

7.1.2 MODE OF TRANSMISSION

The coronavirus infects persons by being transmitted from a particular host to another via aerosol, fomite, or fecal oral route. COVID-19 spreads from people's respiratory droplets and coughing or even sneezing. According to scientists, these respiratory droplets can spread to a distance of about 1.8 meters. In other words, this can infect any individual that is exposed to this [5]. Other studies show that symptomatic individuals tend to be more infected by SARS-CoV-2. The virus is said to survive on steel and plastic surfaces for almost three days. It survives on copper for as long as four days, and on cardboard for 24 hours. The life cycle of the virus in the infected body is recorded. The virus enters the body via the nasal cavity, proceeds to the mucus membranes in the human throat, and becomes entangled to the body. The spikes make the SARS-CoV-2 replicate into various cells in the body. These cells proceed to the bronchial side of the lungs, which leads to damage of the human respiratory tract [6].

7.2 RELATED WORK

Coronavirus-19 is seen as the most concerning global public health problem. Therefore, various scientists/researchers are focused on creating a lasting solution for the menace disease (COVID-19). It was pronounced a pandemic on 13 March 2020. Eden Morales-Narváez and Can Dincer studied the role of biosensing to curb COVID-19. This helped in effective assessment of clinical processes

7.2.1 HISTORY OF SIMILAR PANDEMICS

- **Swine Flu:**
  Swine flu, or swine influenza, can be traced back to the year 1918. It was discovered when swine and humans fell ill at the same time. The influenza

virus was identified after ten years in the year 1930. The strain of the virus was identified from human, swine, and avian, or birds' viruses. The swine flu is regarded as a zoonotic virus [7].

- **Avian flu**:
The avian flu, or avian influenza or bird flu, is a virus that influences birds. This type of flu can be traced to the year 1878, when the first case was recorded. Domestic birds were very affected in developing countries in the 1890s. Recorded millions of birds were dead that year due to the flu.

- **Spanish Flu**:
Researchers and scientists recorded the Spanish flu as the deadliest outbreak in history. It was recorded in the year 1918. It has one of the highest recorded mortality rate in history of about 17 to 50 million. It was observed in the US, UK, France, and Germany [8].

- **Hong Kong Flu**:
Hong Kong flu, as the name implies, is an Asian flu which is one of the major pandemics recorded in the 20th century. The first outbreak was recorded in the year 1968 in Hong Kong (Table 7.3).

7.2.2 VIRUSES OF THE RESPIRATORY TRACT

i. **Influenza Virus**:
The influenza viruses are single-stranded RNA viruses that belong to the family orthomyxoviridae. This kind of virus affects the human respiratory tract. The influenza virus is one of the global pandemics that affect the human respiratory tract. Influenza viruses occur as genetic assortment from hemoglobin and neuraminidase genes. The Avian influenza virus (H5NI), first discovered in Hong Kong in the year 1997, recorded infection of about 18 persons. The number of birds infected was about 1.5 million. However, exposure to infection (from poultry) causes symptoms such as respiratory illnesses [9].

TABLE 7.3
Recorded World Pandemic

Virus	Etiology	Year	Origin
Swine flu	H1N1, H1N2, H2N1, H3N1, H3N2, and H2N3.	1918	USA
Avian flu	H5N1	1957–1958	Singapore
Hong Kong flu	H3N2	1968–1969	Asia
Asian Flu	H2N2	1956	China
MERS	MERS-CoV	2012	Saudi Arabia
SARS	SARS-CoV	2003	Southern China
Ebola Virus	Zaire Ebola	1976	Sudan and Congo

Source: WHO, CDC

ii. **Human Parainfluenza Virus (HPIV)**:

Human parainfluenza virus is a single-stranded DNA that belongs to the family of paramyxoviridae. Parainfluenza virus (PIV) is divided into four (4) serotypes affiliated with human infection. This kind of virus can be detected through immunofluorescent microscopy, cell culture, and polymerase chain-reaction (PCR). Death caused by HPIV globally is rare. Mortality is recorded mostly in the elderly and in toddlers. Human parainfluenza virus has no vaccines yet; however, drugs such as Ribovirin are seen as good potential medications to be administered.

iii. **Adenovirus**:

Adenovirus is a virus that belongs to the family of adenoviridae, with a diameter of 90–100 nm. Adenovirus is a large, non-enveloped virus, with a unique characteristic consisting of spikes. Adenovirus tends to replicate in the nucleus cell of the host using its system. It can be contracted through respiratory droplets. Humans are infected when in contact with the infected person's respiratory droplets. Symptoms could be asymptomatic or severe.

iv. **Coronavirus Disease 2019**:

Coronavirus disease 2019 is a virus that hit global health as a pneumonia case in the Chinese region of Wuhan in December 2019. It was subsequently named SARS-CoV-2 by the International Committee on Taxonomy of Viruses (ICTV) because of the strain of coronavirus traced [10].

- **Classification of COVID-19:** the coronavirus is classified in the family of coronaviridae. It is characterized as alphacoronaviruses and betacoronaviruses. These primarily infect humans. Other traits of coronavirus are the gamma coronavirus and delta coronavirus, which infect apes.

- **Morphology:** the coronavirus has a diameter of about 125 nm. It is characterized by an envelope and spikes sized 85 nm and 20 nm long, respectively. The envelope has a lipid layer which includes the spikes (S), envelope (E), and membrane (M) enclosed with proteins (Figure 7.1).

- **Transmission**:

COVID-19 is transmitted through contact from one infected person to another person via inhaling droplets. This could be through sneezing, singing, and having very close inhalation. When the infected respiratory droplets are dropped on floors and surfaces and subsequently touched by individuals without washing hands, these persons can touch their faces and get infected. The virus can survive on copper for four (4) hours and stay for three (3) days on plastic. Human saliva of an infected person contains heavy presence of the virus within [11].

- **Human metapneumovirus:**

The human metapneumovirus (HMPV) is a single-strand RNA virus that is negative that belongs to the family *Pneumoviridae*. It was first discovered in Holland in the year 2001 using primed Polymerase Chain Reaction. It can be contracted from an infected droplet, fomite, and any secretion.

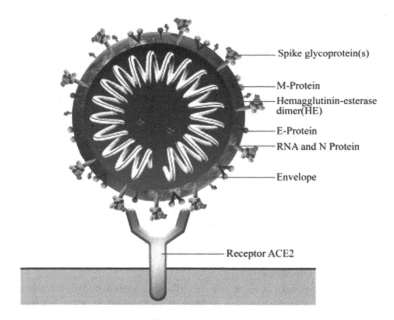

Spike glycoprotein(s)

M-Protein

Hemagglutinin-esterase dimer(HE)

E-Protein

RNA and N Protein

Envelope

Receptor ACE2

FIGURE 7.1   Image of Coronavirus. [Source: Vectormine.com.]

- **Human bocavirus (hBOV)**
  Human bocavirus (hBOV) is a virus of the family *Parvoviridae*.
  This kind of virus is known to infect humans. It was first cloned in
  Karolinska Institute Stockholm, Sweden in 2005.
- **Rhinovirus**
  Rhinoviruses are characterized by their single-strand positive RNA,
  also of a family Picornaviridae. They are symptomatic by common cold
  in humans. It is active in 33–35°C temperature, particularly if found in
  the nostril. The rhinovirus diameter is about 80–120 nm. It was discovered back in 1953 by Johns Hopkins University. Rhinoviruses are
  transmitted through infected respiratory droplets [12].
- **Coronavirus (Cov)**
  Coronavirus is a single-strand positive RNA virus that belongs to the
  family *Coronaviridae*. It is divided into five types as of now. The global
  health problem recorded in 2002 and 2003 was affiliated to SARS-Cov.
  Coronavirus was first discovered in the 1960s in the UK and USA using
  two methods of isolation.

7.3   COVID-19 DIAGNOSIS

The standard test for COVID-19 used by the WHO is the "real-time reverse tran-
scriptase polymerase chain reaction" (rRT – PCR). This method is not only easy to
perform, but also fast. Results can be available two days after testing. The COVID-19

diagnosis uses the nasopharyngeal swab method, which involves the collection of samples through the patient's nose. This sample consists of the collective mixture of saliva and mucus which was collected from the upper respiratory tract. This collection is attained by a cotton swab. The sample is studied in a standard laboratory using the rRT – PCR test. This, subsequently, will determine if the person is infected or not. The nucleic acid amplification test is recommended by the World Health Organization as the used and recognized test for SARS-CoV-2 virus. Another form of diagnosis for COVID-19 is the serological method. This involves the detection of antibodies to fight particular antigens. The serological method is said to lack features to detect COVID-19 at its early embryological stage [13].

7.4 TREATMENT

Drugs: there is no specific medication or vaccine developed to cure COVID-19. However, other drugs developed for similar or other illnesses are reported to exhibit traits that can treat the virus. The World Health Organization, in March 2020, tried another antiviral drug compound that was effective. Numerous drug companies have developed their "possible" treatment. The outlined drugs tested are Hydroxychloroquine, Remdesivir, and alcohol. Drugs such as the Shuang-Huang-Lian (SHL) were also considered to treat COVID-19. This is a Chinese traditional drug effective in treating bacterial infections [14].

I. **Vaccine:** researchers are focused on building a vaccine for COVID-19. There is no vaccine for now, but researchers are interested in using previous studies related to SARS-CoV. Some vaccines developed for SARS-CoV and used as trial vaccines for COVID-19 are:

- **Johnson & Johnson vaccine:** Johnson & Johnson's COVID-19 lead vaccine was developed on 30 March 2020, identified after 90 days of extensive research of different vaccine in afflation with the Israeli Beth Deconess Medical Center. Johnson & Johnson's COVID-19 lead vaccine has the ability to develop new vaccines. This vaccine is planned to begin its human clinical trials by September 2020. Johnson & Johnson is working with the Biomedical Advance Research and Development Authority (BARDA) on the COVID-19 vaccine [15].
- **Cansino's Ads-nCoV:** Ads-nCoV is the adenovirus type-5 vector-based vaccine of COVID-19 developed by Cansino Biological Inc in an affiliation with the Beijing Institute of Technology (BIT) [16].
- **Pittsburgh coronavirus vaccine:** Pittcovaccis a coronavirus vaccine developed by Pittsburgh School of Medicine researchers. The vaccine is developed against SARS-CoV-2. It was used to test its potentials on mice, however, it helped in the growth of antibodies against the virus (SARS-CoV-2) after 14 days of usage [17] (Table 7.4).

II. **Drugs:**

- **Dexamethasone:** this antiviral drug was reported to be effective against COVID-19 on 16 June 2020. Dexamethasone was said to be impactful

TABLE 7.4
Vaccines Used for COVID-19

Vaccine Type	Vaccine Title	Vaccine Sponsor
Adenovirus type-5 vector	Adenovirus coronavirus 2019-nCoV is a randomized, placebo-controlled, and double blinded vaccine.	Academy of Military Medical Sciences, Institute of Biotechnology.
mRNA	Vaccine against COVID-2019 used as trial.	BioNTech RNA pharmaceuticals GmbH.
Inactivated +Alum	Inactivated vaccine with prophylaxis against COVID-19.	Sinovac research and development, Sinovac Biotech Ltd.
ChAdOX1	Research on COVID-19 vaccine.	Oxford University UK
Electroporation DNA plasmid vaccine	Tolerable and safe for COVID-19.	Inovio pharmaceuticals

Source: WHO Draft Landscape of COVID-19 Vaccines – 26 April 2020

TABLE 7.5
Tested Drugs Used in COVID-19 Treatment

Drug	Title	Sponsor
Remdesivir	Used in evaluating activeness of Remdesivir (Gs-574^{tm}) in COVID-19.	Gilead sciences
Favipiravir	Favipiravir used in severe COVID-19 patients (FIC).	Shahid Beheshi University of Medical Sciences.
Hydroxychloroquine with Azithromycin	Azithromycin in hospitalized COVID-19 patients (AIC).	Shahid Beheshi University of Medical sciences.
Tocilizumab	Tested on COVID-19 patients.	Massachussetts General Hospital.
Dexamethasone	Antiviral drug against COVID-19 patients used in hospitalized patients on ventilator.	National Health service UK.
Loinavir/Ritonavir	Effective in treating COVID-19 patients in Colombia.	Universidad nacional de colombia

US National Library of Medicine (Trial phases as on 29 April)

on reduced mortality rate related to COVID-19 with patients on ventilators. The patients were on dexamethasone, 6 mg dosage, once per day (intravenous or oral administered). This was observed for ten days in comparison with 4,321 patients not on the dosage. Patients that received dexamethasone were said to have survived. WHO recommended dexamethasone drugs as a treatment to reduce the death rate in COVID-19 patients [18] (Table 7.5).

7.5 PREVENTION

Preventive measures against COVID-19 are very important in curtailing COVID-19.

- **Sanitation:** sanitation is one crucial step to control the spread of COVID-19. Hands should be kept clean. This is done with water and soap or sanitizer.
- **Social distancing:** social distancing of about 3 feet (1 meter) from other humans should be observed. In other words, social distancing could be practiced by staying at home.
- **Face mask/hand gloves:** face masks and hand gloves are used in public places to prevent the spread of COVID-19. These materials are advised to be dumped appropriately [19] (Figure 7.2).

7.6 INTERNET OF THINGS AND INTERNET OF MATERIAL THINGS (IOT AND IOMT)

This process connects software application and medical devices with the health care IT system. The internet is connected and tends to make things easier. IoT and IoMT are important in collecting, analyzing, and transmitting patient data to the health

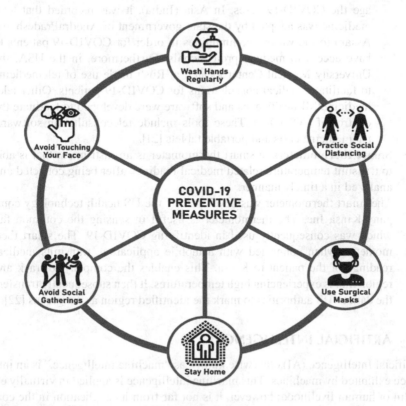

FIGURE 7.2 Preventive measures for COVID-19.

care system efficiently. This process is applied to control the spread of COVID-19 [20]. The IoT and IoMT technologies involved in the control and management of the spread of COVID-19 include:

- **Telemedicine:** telemedicine is an act of monitoring a patient's medical record using IoMT technology to help patients that are not connected to medical services. This method is essential in the control of COVID-19. Online medical consultations have been recorded since the inception of this terrible outbreak of COVID-19. Doctors and other paramedics in other parts of the world have made medical consultations available via telehealth. This process was recorded in the office of civil rights (OCR) and with the centers for Medicare and medic services (CMS) in the USA. Telemedicine techniques are important in the telehealth control of COVID-19 in two great ways:
  (i)   Telemedicine has greatly lowered the spread of the COVID-19 virus from host persons to uninfected persons.
  (ii) Telemedicine has reduced the workload of other medical professionals that should be at work taking care of infected persons.
        Telemedicine has been adopted in different parts of the world to manage the COVID-19 cases. In Asia (India), it was recorded that telemedicine was adopted by the state government of AnddraPradesh and Assam to the various communities in order for COVID-19 patients to have access to medical professionals. Furthermore, in the USA, the University Medical Center located at Rush made use of telemedicine to facilitate medical consultations for COVID-19 patients. Other telemedicine/MLhealth apps and software were developed to facilitate the control of COVID-19. These tools include teleconsultation software, telemedicine carts and portable tablets [21].
- **Smart thermometers**: a smart thermometer is an instrument that is able to transmit temperature related medical readings after being collected and analyzed in a timely manner.
  The smart thermometer was developed by the US health technology company Kinsa Inc. The thermometer is useful in sensing the common flu, which was consequently used in identifying COVID-19. The smart thermometer, when connected with a mobile application, transmits medical readings of the patient to Kinsa. This enables the company to track any region that is experiencing high temperatures. It then subsequently transfers the data to US authorities to mark the identified region as dangerous [22].

7.7   ARTIFICIAL INTELLIGENCE

Artificial Intelligence (AI),otherwise known as "machine intelligence," is an intelligence exhibited by machines. This machine intelligence is applied in virtually every realm of human livelihood; however, it is not far from its application in the control and management of the COVID-19 outbreak [23]. This includes different ways:

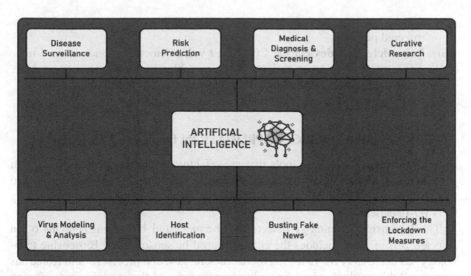

FIGURE 7.3 Artificial Intelligence application for COVID-19.

- **Surveillance:** the COVID-19 surveillance was done by BlueDot, a health surveillance company based in Toronto, Canada. This company was able to identify potential COVID-19 spread in December 2019.

  Furthermore, other similar companies evolved using AI to forecast the risk affiliated with this disease.
- **Disease prediction:** disease prediction enables forecasting the risk associated with COVID-19. This risk could be the risk involved in getting infected and prediction of the risk involved in having symptoms, or prediction of the risk of getting treated using a particular stereotyped method when infected (patient). However, artificial intelligence is applied to determine the survival probability and the treatment involved for COVID-19 infected persons [24] (Figure 7.3).

7.8 DIAGNOSIS AND SCREENING

COVID-19 is diagnosed rapidly to curtail the spread of the virus. Artificial Intelligence tools are used in the diagnosis. This enables the availability of medical diagnosis and screening as a result of shortage in testing kits worldwide [25]. Artificial Intelligence (AI) screening and diagnosis processes involve:

(i) **Medical imaging:** this involves the application of AI in image-based medical diagnosis. Radiologists use the topography scans and X-rays using Artificial Intelligence to diagnose COVID-19 patients.
(ii) **Facial scanners:** face scanners are used in the screening of the infected persons with COVID-19. These scanners are the IR temperature, which is used to screen people for high temperature. Currently, these face

scanners are adopted using Artificial Intelligence cameras to track any infected person.

(iii) **Voice detection device:** the COVID-19 voice detection device is used in difficult times to screen patients. This is enabled by the application of AI in the diagnosis. It detects the different strains of the virus and accurately diagnoses COVID-19 patients using algorithms and AI devices [26].

7.9   BIOSENSING DEVICES APPLICATION IN COVID-19 PATIENTS

Biosensors are strong testing tools that are effective in clinical processes and that give broad solutions to the patient's wellbeing through the level of damage caused by the virus or infection. In other words, the biosensing devices are used for testing COVID-19 patients.

The biosensing technology detects the chemical and biological contents of an infected person. This includes the enzyme-based biosensors [27]. Biosensing technology has made COVID-19 testing more efficient, fast, and precise. South Korea has introduced this method, which has subsequently reduced the mortality rate after an organized test known as "phone booth" test. Furthermore, Germany is also engaged in a sensitization outreach target of testing about 400,000 COVID-19 patients per week. These processes are no doubt able to reduce the death rate of the mentioned places.

I. **Polymerase chain reaction:** the PCR test is important in the "tracing and isolating" of patients. The genetic code of COVID-19 has been published in January 2020 by a People's Republic of China-based scientist. The PCR-based test has been adopted in China and many parts of the world to diagnose, using the gold-standard method. The polymerase chain reaction involves the virus [28].

II. **CRISPR technology:** clustered regularly interspaced short palindromic repeats (CRISPR) is a technology applied in gene editing science. In other words, CRISPR is a "promising and powerful tool" (described by Li et al., 2019) that is used in DNA sequencing that could be found in unicellular organisms (prokaryotes), which could be bacteria and archae. Furthermore, CRISPR-cas enzymes are programmed to be effective by CRISPR RNAs or single-guide RNAs (SgRNAs) that target nucleic acids in bacteria, viruses (including COVID-19), and cancer. Scientists and researchers globally are working on developing affordable, easy and sensitive devices that are highly efficient. This led to developing the CRISPR-Cas system [29]. CRISPR-Cas has two main approaches, the binding-based CRISPR and cleavage-based.

• **Mammoth detection:** the Mammoth detection was employed using the Cas-12 enzyme, which targets single-stranded RNAs and DNAs. Mammoth Biosciences was used in detecting about ten or more copies per µL used for fluorescence detection of SARS-COV-2 virus genome, within a scope of about 40 minutes. This method happens when E and N genes are extracted from the patient swab [30].

- **Sherlock detection:** the Sherlock detection method was used by Feng Zhang to detect COVID-19 with a detection limit recorded of about "10 and 100 copies per µL." This method is determined in less than an hour using the recombinase and the Cas 13 enzyme [31].
- **Sensor material (substrates) detection:** This method functions using the recombinant viral antigen and the immunoglobulins and is used to detect the presence of COVID-19 in the blood. The sensor material method is employed in "home-pregnancy test," or otherwise known as ovulation tests. This method is said to be "safe and user-friendly." It is also approved and used in places such as Germany, the USA, Australia, Singapore, and China. SARS-COV-2 can be detected using these devices by placing the patient's blood, serum or plasma for infection analysis, and the results could be ready within a period of 15 minutes [32].
- **CoNVaT project detection:** the CoNVaT project is a European research and development system that puts rapid effort to counter the COVID-19 pandemic.
  The optical technology project is said to be a "unique biosensor." This method of biosensing can test the saliva and nasal samples of the patient and can detect whether a minor strain of the virus is present. The CoNVaT detection is aimed to expand its scope of detection of COVID-19 in virus-carrying organisms such as bats [33].

7.10 CLOUD COMPUTING USED IN COVID-19

Machine learning and cloud computing models are designed to predict an accurate number of COVID-19 new cases and the dates that this may occur. This method gives safe computation and fast data analysis. The cloud computing system enables hospitals to have records of infected persons. These include getting the patients median and average population density, health facilities, and weather conditions of the place. Other methods of cloud computing recorded in COVID-19 include the single core Azure B1s virtual machines and 1-GiB RAM. HealthFog was also recorded to have numerous analyses to predict metrics used to manage patients. Hitherto, specialists predicted the booming period for the cloud technology. This prediction resulted in the COVID-19 pandemic impact on the cloud technology as a result of the pandemic [34] (Figure 7.4 and Table 7.6).

7.11 INTERNET OF THINGS USED IN COVID-19

Internet of Things (IoT) technology has been used for information and survellance during the pandemic. This technology is used in tackling various challenges during the quarantine period.

The use of IoT is recorded to have reduced costs in healthcare and also improved treatment of infected persons. The Internet of Things (IoT) is known as digital computing tactics and mechanical processes that transmit data through a network without

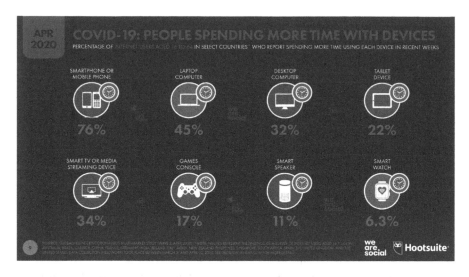

FIGURE 7.4   IoT and cloud computing during the COVID-19 period.

TABLE 7.6
Comparison among the Different Technologies Used in COVID-19 Patients

Technology	Method	Sponsors
CRISPR technology	CRISPR-Cas 12, Cas 13 based-biosensing technology is used in genome in COVID-19 Patients.	Doudna Lab, University of California Berkeley, Mammoth Biosciences.
Mammoth detection technique	SARS-CoV DETECTR used in detecting COVID-19.	Developed by UC San Francisco and Mammoth Biosciences.
Sherlock detection technique	SHERLOCK method used to test COVID-19 patients using RNA purified sample.	SHERLOCK Biosciences. Zhang Lab.
DETECTRE technique	Simple and efficient method used in detecting nucleic acids, including COVID-19.	Mammoth Biosciences.
Sensor material detection technique	Used in detecting SARS-COV-2 using Field-effect transistor (FET).	Biosensor Lab for Field-effect transistor (FET).
Artificial Intelligence	Used in surveillance, disease prediction, diagnosis and screening..	BlueDot Company, Toronto, Canada.
CoNVaT project Detection	Optical biosensor, detects COVID-19 in 30 minutes.	Catalan Institute of Nanoscience and Nanotechnology.
IoM and IoT technology	Digital computing technique.	Centers for Medicare and medics (USA).
Cloud computing	Used as computing models.	HealthFog.

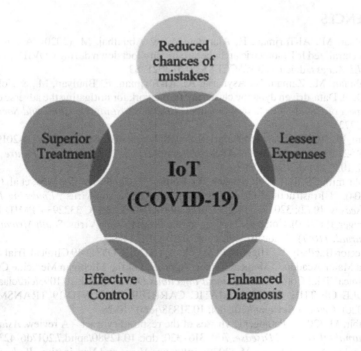

FIGURE 7.5   Application of IoT for COVID-19.

human effort. IoT is also used against the pandemic (COVID-19) in countries such as India. IoT is connected with different network systems such as software, hardware, network and computer. It has been able to help patients to be aware of the virus. The advantage of the Internet of Things is that, it has identified infected persons and monitored them. Areas and persons of high-risk are identified through the Internet-based network system [35] (Figure 7.5).

7.12 CONCLUSION

The inception of the COVID-19 outbreak has open numerous alternatives and ways to curtail the virus using medicine and technology. These methods have been recorded to be eligible to manage COVID-19 virus. This research focused on using technology such as IOT, AI, Biosensor, and CRISPR-Cas detection processes to manage the virus.

The integration of these tools is recorded to be effective in studies compiled. We accessed the mechanism, mode of transmission, and diagnosis of the virus in its different forms. Preventive measures are analyzed using basic healthcare system. The treatment of the virus is vital at this moment; companies, researchers, institutions, and laboratories are designing ways to curb this virus. Primarily, this research focuses on using technologies such as IoT, CRISPR detection, AI, and Biosensor detection methods to manage the COVID-19 pandemic using different affiliated studies.

REFERENCES

1. Kolhar, M., Al-Turjman, F., Alameen, A., & Abualhaj, M. (2020). A three layered decentralized IoT biometric architecture for city lockdown during COVID-19 outbreak. *IEEE Access*. doi: 10.1109/ACCESS.2020.3021983

2. Rahman, M., Zaman, N., Asyharia, A., Al-Turjman, F., Bhuiyan, M., & Zolkipli, M. (2020). Data-driven dynamic clustering framework for mitigating the adverse economic impact of Covid-19 lockdown practices. *Elsevier Sustainable Cities and Societies*, 62, 102372.

3. Fani, M., Teimoori, A., & Ghafari, S. (2020). Comparison of the COVID-2019 (SARS-CoV-2) pathogenesis with SARS-CoV and MERS-CoV infections. *Future Virology*. doi: 10.2217/fvl-2020-0050

4. Goldsmith CS, Tatti KM, Ksiazek TG, Rollin PE, Comer JA, Lee WW, et al. (February 2004). "Ultrastructural characterization of SARS coronavirus". *Emerging Infectious Diseases*. **10** (2): 320–26. doi:10.3201/eid1002.030913. PMC 3322934. PMID 15030705

5. Kruger, P. (2020). Compelled testing for the novel Corona Virus. *South African Medical Journal*, *110*(7), 0. doi: 10.7196/samj.2020.v110i7.14890

6. Spector-Bagdady, K., Higgins, P., & Lok, A. (2020). COVID-19 Clinical Trial Oversight at a Major Academic Medical Center: Approach of the Michigan Medicine COVID-19 Clinical Trial Committees. *Clinical Infectious Diseases*. doi: 10.1093/cid/ciaa560

7. ROLE OF THE ASYMPTOMATIC CARRIER IN COVID-19 TRANSMISSION. (2020). *Critical Review*, 7(10). doi: 10.31838/jcr.07.10.28

8. Kabir, M. (2017). Pathogenic viruses of the respiratory tract – A review. *Asian Pacific Journal Of Tropical Disease*, *7*(5), 316–320. doi: 10.12980/apjtd.7.2017d6-423

9. Nogales, A., & DeDiego, M. (2020). Influenza Virus and Vaccination. *Pathogens*, *9*(3), 220. doi: 10.3390/pathogens9030220

10. Carter, B. (2020). My Pathway to Adeno-Associated Virus and Adeno-Associated Virus Gene Therapy: A Personal Perspective. *Human Gene Therapy*, *31*(9–10), 494–498. doi: 10.1089/hum.2020.29120.bca

11. Barupal, T., Tak, P., & Meena, M. (2020). COVID-19: Morphology, Characteristics, Symptoms, Prevention, Clinical Diagnosis and Current Scenario. *Coronaviruses*, *01*. doi: 10.2174/2666796701999200617161348

12. Stobart, C., Nosek, J., & Moore, M. (2017). Rhinovirus Biology, Antigenic Diversity, and Advancements in the Design of a Human Rhinovirus Vaccine. *Frontiers In Microbiology*, 8. doi: 10.3389/fmicb.2017.02412

13. Hodinka R. (2016) Respiratory RNA viruses. *Microbiology Spectrum* 2016; doi:10.1128/microbiolspec.DMIH2-0028-2016.

14. The hunt for an effective treatment for COVID-19. (2020). *The Pharmaceutical Journal*. doi: 10.1211/pj.2020.20207883

15. Race for a COVID-19 vaccine. (2020). *Ebiomedicine*, *55*, 102817. doi: 10.1016/j.ebiom.2020.102817

16. Efficacy and Safety of Hydroxychloroquine for Treatment of Pneumonia Caused by 2019-nCoV (HC-nCoV). (2020). *Case Medical Research*. doi: 10.31525/ct1-nct04261517

17. Kim, E., Erdos, G., Huang, S., Kenniston, T., Balmert, S., & Carey, C. et al. (2020). Microneedle array delivered recombinant coronavirus vaccines: Immunogenicity and rapid translational development. *Ebiomedicine*, *55*, 102743. doi: 10.1016/j.ebiom.2020.102743

18. Dexamethasone is 'first drug' to be shown to improve survival in COVID-19. (2020). *The Pharmaceutical Journal*. doi: 10.1211/pj.2020.20208074

19. Escher, A., 2020. An ounce of prevention: Coronavirus (COVID-19) and mass gatherings. *Cureus*,.

20. Menon, V., Jacob, S., Joseph, S., Sehdev, P., Khosravi, M. and Al-Turjman, F., 2020. An IoT-enabled intelligent automobile system for smart cities. *Internet of Things*, p.100213.
21. Kannampallil, T., & Ma, J., 2020. Digital Translucence: Adapting Telemedicine Delivery Post-COVID-19. *Telemedicine and e-Health*,.
22. Toh, C., & Webb, W., 2020. The Smart City and Covid-19. *IET Smart Cities*,.
23. Tárnok, A., 2020. Machine Learning, COVID-19 (2019-nCoV), and multi-OMICS. *Cytometry. Part A*, 97(3), pp.215–216.
24. Challener, D., Dowdy, S., & O'Horo, J., 2020. Mayo Clinic Strategies for COVID-19 Analytics and Prediction Modeling During the COVID-19 Pandemic. *Mayo Clinic Proceedings*,.
25. Cho, A., 2020. Artificial intelligence systems aim to sniff out signs of COVID-19 outbreaks. *Science*,.
26. Kong, W., & Agarwal, P., 2020. Chest Imaging Appearance of COVID-19 Infection. *Radiology: Cardiothoracic Imaging*, 2(1), p.e200028.
27. Morales-Narváez, E., & Dincer, C., 2020. The impact of biosensing in a pandemic outbreak: COVID-19. *Biosensors and Bioelectronics*, 163, p.112274.
28. Elkattawy, S., Younes, I., & Noori, M., 2020. A Case Report of Polymerase Chain Reaction-Confirmed COVID-19 in a Patient With Right Ventricular Thrombus and Bilateral Deep Vein Thrombosis. *Cureus*,.
29. Tsang, J., & LaManna, C., 2020. Open Sharing During COVID-19: CRISPR-Based Detection Tools. *The CRISPR Journal*, 3(3), pp.142–145.
30. *International Journal of Innovative Technology and Exploring Engineering*, 2020. Performance Result for Detection of COVID-19 using Deep Learning. 9(7), pp.699–703.
31. *MEDICC Review*, 2020. COVID-19 Case Detection: Cuba's Active Screening Approach. 22(2), p.58.
32. *Clinical OMICs*, 2019. Sherlock Biosciences Raises $31M for CRISPR Dx Development. 6(3), pp.7–7.
33. Sberna, G., Amendola, A., Valli, M., Carletti, F., Capobianchi, M., Bordi, L., & Lalle, E., (2020). Trend of respiratory pathogens during the COVID-19 epidemic. *Journal of Clinical Virology*, 129, p.104470.
34. Tuli, S., Tuli, S., Tuli, R., & Gill, S. (2020). Predicting the growth and trend of COVID-19 pandemic using machine learning and cloud computing. *Internet Of Things*, 11, 100222. doi: 10.1016/j.iot.2020.100222
35. Waheed, A., Goyal, M. , Gupta, D. , Khanna, A., Al-Turjman, F., Pinheiro, P. R. (2020). CovidGAN: Data augmentation using auxiliary classifier GAN for improved Covid-19 detection. *IEEE Access*. doi: 10.1109/ACCESS.2020.2994762

8 How Artificial Intelligence and IoT Aid in Fighting COVID-19

Abdullahi Umar Ibrahim, Mehmet Ozsoz,
Fadi Al-Turjman, Pwadubashiyi Pwavodi Coston,
and Basil Bartholomew Duwa

CONTENTS

8.1 INTRODUCTION

The outbreak of the novel coronavirus 2019 has taken the world by storm, spreading to almost every part of the world. The word "pandemic" was introduced in 2005 by the World Health Organization (WHO) as an epidemic affecting the globe or many areas, or disease that spread or cross to many countries and thus affecting large number of populations. So far, pandemics of disease have been declared five times, including the influenza pandemic in 2009, Polio in 2014, Ebola in 2014 and 2019, Zika virus in 2016, and COVID-19 in 2020. Prior to the outbreak of COVID-19, other viral pathogens have raised international concerns, such as Zika and Ebola viruses, along with viruses from the same family as COVID-19, which include severe acute respiratory syndrome coronavirus (SARS-CoV) in 2002 and Middle East respiratory syndrome coronavirus (MERS-CoV) in 2012 (Fan et al., 2019; Paules et al., 2020; Ul Qamar et al., 2020).

The first case of COVID-19 was reported in Wuhan City, mainland China, on new year's eve, and the number escalated to over three million confirmed cases and a death toll of close to 300 thousand. The pandemic has caused many setbacks as well as global economic impacts as a result of lockdowns, quarantines, flight and events cancelations, schools, market, border closures and suspension of routine, religious, social, and sport activities. Many businesses have reported financial losses of billions of dollars, a crash of the crude oil market and an increase in the unemployment rate (Paules et al. 2020).

Medical experts, governments, and security agencies have been working together to prevent the continuous outbreak of COVID-19 through diagnosis based on testing and screening, treatment, social distancing, self-isolation, and the restriction of movements. However, the battalions of artificial intelligence and IoT have been on the warfront as tools for fighting against the widespread diagnosis and identification of drugs that can be used for the treatment of COVID-19.

The application of artificial intelligence and machine learning is transforming the field of medicine and the health care sectors. Scientist employ machine learning models to detect patterns in data related to diseases, which involves the prediction of diseases through transmission and genomics, identification of drugs that can be used to treat different diseases, as well as analysis of data and management of hospital records (Miotto et al., 2018; Naylor, 2018).

8.1.1 SCOPE

This chapter aims to offer insight on Coronaviruses and the use of IoT- and artificial intelligence-driven tools for detection, prediction, and identification of drugs and vaccines. We highlighted the strains, transmission, and symptoms of coronaviruses in Section 8.2. In Section 8.3, we overview the general use of IoT- and artificial intelligence-driven tools for detection, prediction, and identification of drugs and vaccines against coronaviruses

8.2 CORONAVIRUS PANDEMIC

Corona virus is a single-stranded RNA virus which has a feature of being spherical or pleomorphic and covered with glycoprotein, which is club-shaped. This virus has four different sub-types, which are alpha, beta, gamma, and delta, and each has different serotypes, with symptoms seen to affect both humans and animals (Kumar et al., 2020).

Coronavirus was first discovered in the 1960s, and in 2001, a Canadian study showed that approximately 500 patients were identified with the virus with flu-like symptoms (Kumar et al., 2020). The virus was then treated as a non-fatal virus until 2002 and 2003, when reports showed that there was a wide spread of the virus to many countries as a severe acute respiratory syndrome (SARS-CoV) (Cui et al., 2019). A decade later, there was an outbreak of Middle East Respiratory Syndrome (MERS), which was found to be caused by the MERS-CoV (Khan et al.) (4,5). COVID-19 was first discovered in Wuhan, China, and this virus presented symptoms of pneumonia in the patients affected by it (Khan et al., 2020).

This virus is known to be contagious from person to person through airborne zoonotic droplets that affect the respiratory system and the digestive system, as shown in Figure 8.1. In 2019, a study was published stating that the Angiotensin converting enzyme 2 (ACE2) receptor is used by the virus to gain entry into human cells (Lekto and Munster, 2020; Kumar et al., 2020). According to reports published on the 24 January 2020, all patients infected with the coronavirus present the same features, such as cough, fever, fatigue, and other uncommon features based on the system of the patient (Chan et al., 2020; Huang et al., 2020).

There is presently no cure or vaccine, but researchers and scientists around the world are working to discover how to prevent it and even cure it with vaccines. WHO and ECDC have given some guidelines on how to prevent its transmission from person to person (Kumar et al., 2020). Doctors and researchers are doing their best to find a proper solution to this virus. There is no special vaccine for treating it yet, rather, supportive therapy is given to manage the condition (Zhao et al., 2003; Chan et al., 2013).

Laboratory diagnosis include clinical specimens of nasal secretions, blood, sputum and bronchoalveolar lavage used for molecular and serological tests. Molecular tests are based on real-time PCR or northern blotting, and serological tests are based on ELISA or western blots (Zu et al., 2020; Li et al., 2020).

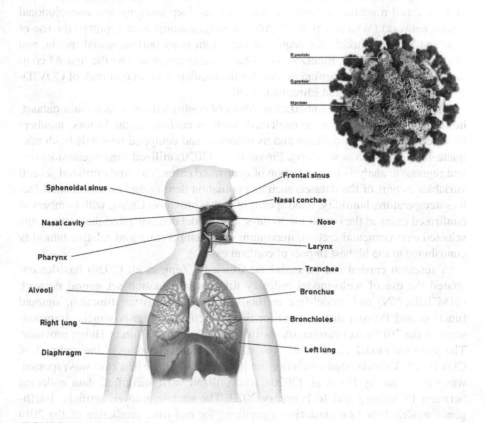

FIGURE 8.1 Transmission of coronavirus.

8.3 APPLICATION OF ARTIFICIAL INTELLIGENCE

8.3.1 PREDICTION

As the number of confirmed cases increases globally, prediction of continuous spread is highly required in order to take preventative measures. The application of artificial intelligence in the healthcare sector is gradually transforming the sector due to its broad application in the detection of diseases, clinical diagnosis, drug discovery, and analysis of medical records. The use of AI-driven tools is aiding epidemiologist for prediction of outbreak and screening of potential drugs against newly discovered diseases. One of the challenges faced by medical experts is acquiring actual numbers of cases as a general dataset. Moreover, the use of artificial intelligence models can assist epidemiologist and data analysts in collecting the evolving data and performing further analysis for decision (Fan et al., 2019; Long & Ehrenfeld, 2020).

The use of prediction models along with several features and variables is significantly aiding in estimating or forecasting the number of people that may contract the disease, and thus could help medical experts in taking measures, in the allocation of healthcare facilities, and the screening process. There is a wide range of prediction models reported in the literature, such as traditional machine learning algorithms and advanced machine learning models (such as deep learning and convolutional neural network) (Wynants et al., 2020). Recently, scientist have reported the use of machine learning models for acquiring data from news outlets, social media, and other sources. However, BlueDot, an AI-based company, is among the first AI companies to use machine learning models for the prediction of an outbreak of COVID-19 prior to 2020 (Long and Ehrenfeld, 2020).

Many published articles utilized numbers of confirmed cases as a main dataset, however, other variables were neglected, such as environmental factors, numbers of tested people in a population and its outcome, and equipped hospitals (with adequate facilities, such ventilators). Pirouz et al. (2020) utilized binary classification and regression analysis for prediction of confirmed cases. The study utilized several variables as part of the dataset, such as population density and environmental factors (temperature, humidity, wind speed) of Hubei province, China, with numbers of confirmed cases as the output for 30 days. The model demonstrated that, among the selected environmental factors, maximum daily temperature and relative humidity contributed to the highest impact of confirm cases.

A research carried out on mainland China by Zeng et al. (2020) has demonstrated the use of multi-model ordinary differential equation set neural network (MMODEs-NN) and model-free methods (based on Gaussian function, sigmoid function, and Poisson distribution) for the prediction of inter-provincial transmissions of the 2019 novel coronavirus with high regard from China's Hubei province. The proposed model has shown a consistent and realistic ending of the outbreak of COVID-19. A similar studied carried out in China, where the first case was reported, was carried out by Hu et al. (2020), who utilized WHO-acquired data collected between 19 January and 16 February 2020. The study employed artificial intelligence models based on clustering algorithms for real-time prediction of the 2019 novel coronavirus outbreak within China, based on size estimation, lengths, and ending time of the outbreak. The model was successful in predicting the trajectory of the 2019 novel coronavirus by clustering cities.

The allocation of resources and prediction of patients that could be at risk of developing acute respiratory distress syndrome (ARDS) are very critical in controlling and preventing COVID-19 pandemic. In order to provide rapid, clinical decision-making support for clinicians and epidemiologists, Jiang et al. (2020) utilized artificial intelligence techniques with a predictive analytics ability, using real patient data acquired from two different hospital in China. The artificial intelligence models achieved 80% and 70% accuracy in the prediction of severe cases based on historical data of patients.

8.3.2 DETECTION OF COVID-19 USING ARTIFICIAL INTELLIGENCE MODELS

Real-time polymerase chain reaction (RT-PCR) is currently the gold standard method used by medical laboratory technologies for the detection of COVID-19 in patient samples based on nucleic acid (i.e. RNA for viruses) (Li et al., 2020). Medical test kits are currently available worldwide. However, long protocol to install and run the test, false results, and high cost are some of the challenges of using the medical kits. In order to develop an alternative or confirmatory test, scientist turn to artificial intelligence techniques.

Datasets are one of the critical components in artificial intelligence. Large amounts of datasets enables AI models to learn patterns effectively and to increase generatability. The research published by Wang et al. (2020) utilized 453 total CT scan images of confirmed cases of COVID-19 acquired from patients that were previously diagnosed with viral pneumonia. The 453 images are partitioned into 217 images for training, using an inception migration-learning model, and 236 for validation and testing. Even though the research utilized a lesser amount of data, the model was able to achieve an external testing accuracy of 73.1%, sensitivity of 74%, and specificity of 67%, and an internal validation accuracy of 82.9%, sensitivity of 84%, and specificity of 80.5%. However, more datasets are required to enable the model to make accurate predictions and increase generality.

Differentiating between viral strains that caused pneumonia is significant for the detection of COVID-19 in patient CT scan images. The study by Gozes et al. (2020) confronted the stated challenge by developing an artificial intelligence-based automated detection model using CT images, as well as tracking and quantification of COVID-19. The study utilized multiple datasets acquired from China and the USA. The dataset was partitioned into training and testing and trained using robust 2D and 3D deep learning models. The results have shown the models achieved high AUC value, sensitivity, and specificity.

Many approaches developed their models from scratch. However, the use of transfer learning has been shown to increase efficiency of models for classification of objects. Apostolopoulos and Mpesiana (2020) utilized transfer learning models of VGG19, MobileNet v2, Xception, Inception, and Inception ResNet v2 trained to classify patients with COVID-19 disease, bacterial pneumonia, and health patients. The study utilized 2 datasets; (1) 1427 total X-ray images (504 images of healthy patients, 700 images of confirmed bacterial pneumonia and 224 images of confirmed COVID-19 disease. (2) 1442 total X-ray images (504 images of healthy patients, 714 images of confirmed bacterial pneumonia and 224 images of confirmed COVID-19 disease. The result has shown MobileNet v2, achieved higher accuracy, sensitivity, and specificity of 96.78%, 98.66%, and 96.46% respectively (Figure 8.2).

While many published articles utilized CT scans images for classification of COVID-19, other research adopted other parameters based on symptoms related to COVID-19. A study by Maghdid et al. (2020) demonstrated how artificial intelligence models can be used for detection of COVID-19 using smartphones equipped with powerful tools such as rich processors, memory space, and sensors based on inertial sensors, wireless chipsets/sensors, humidity sensors, and temperature sensors. The methodology is based on the use of AI-driven models which read signals assimilated from sensors to predict the grade of severity of the pneumonia, which constitutes the major symptom or parameter for diagnosis of COVID-19.

Viral pneumonia is caused by different strains of viruses. In order to distinguish between some of these strains, Xu et al. (2020) utilized artificial intelligence models to distinguish between COVID-19, Influenza-A viral pneumonia, and healthy cases

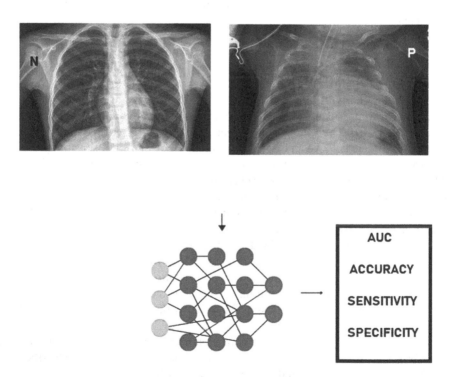

FIGURE 8.2 The use of artificial intelligence tools for the classification of COVID-19 disease. N: Negative, P: Positive, AUC: Area under the curve.

acquired from positive and negative patient's computed tomography (CT) images. The research utilized 618 total CT scans images, 219 images from 110 patients with COVID-19, 224 CT images from 224 patients with the Influenza-A virus, and 175 CT images from healthy people. The images were trained using a 3-dimensional deep learning model and the result achieved an overall accuracy of 86.7%.

8.3.3 Identification of Potential Vaccines Using Artificial Intelligence

Artificial intelligence is one such innovation that can undoubtedly stop the spread of the COVID-19; it recognizes the high-hazard patients and is valuable in controlling this disease continuously. It can likewise anticipate the chance of mortality by dissecting past information of the patients. Artificial intelligence can assist us with fighting this infection by populace screening, clinical assistance, warning, and recommendations about disease control (Vaishya et al., 2020).

Artificial intelligence is utilized for sedate research by investigating the accessible information on COVID-19. It is valuable for medicating conveyance plans and advancement. This innovation is utilized in accelerating drug testing progressively, where standard testing takes a lot of time and consequently assists with quickening this procedure essentially, which may not be conceivable by a human (Haleem et al., 2019). It can assist in recognizing valuable medications for the treatment of COVID-19 patients. It has become an amazing asset for analytic test structures and immunization advancement (Sohrabi et al., 2020).

Different systems are being tried in China, including drug repurposing. A pretrained deep learning-based drug-target interaction model, termed Molecule Transformer-Drug Target Interaction (MT-DTI), was utilized to distinguish industrially accessible medications that could follow up on viral proteins of SARS-CoV-2. Atazanavir, an antiretroviral prescription used to treat and forestall the human immunodeficiency infection (HIV), was analyzed as the best substance (Luo et al., 2020).

Kandeel and Al-Nazawi, (2020) used the first resolved COVID-19 crystal structure targeted in a virtual screening study approved by FDA drugs dataset. The current research gave an extensive focus on the COVID-19 structure of Mpro and found reasonable spare medications for repurposing against the viral Mpro. Ribavirin, telbivudine, nutrient B12, and nicotinamide can be joined and utilized for COVID treatment.

These mentioned drugs are recorded as safe medications for potential treatment of the COVID-19 virus. In other words, Zhavoronko (2020), used deep learning methodology in regenerative science as a tool to control and manage the Virus, respectively. These processes can be elaborated to different fields relating to regenerative sciences, which also include affiliated techniques in handling the virus such as in artificial intelligence and a computer-based knowledge such as the machine learning method to control COVID-19 virus.

In another similar research, high-throughput screening was done as a way to screen the potential COVID sedate, utilizing a dataset of groupings and structures of SARS-CoV. This was driven from PDB database, utilizing NCBI-impact v2.9, introduced on a framework and other molecules from Drug bank (Zhou et al., 2020).

Imaging isn't shown in patients with suspected COVID-19 and mellow clinical highlights, except if they are exposed to danger of the illness. Imaging is demonstrated in a patient with COVID-19 and exacerbating respiratory status. In an asset-obliged condition, imaging is demonstrated for clinical triage of patients with suspected COVID-19 who present with moderate-extreme clinical highlights and a high pre-test likelihood of illness (Li et al., 2020).

Artificial intelligence is an up-and-coming valuable device to recognize early contaminations due to coronavirus. Furthermore, it helps in observing the state of affected patients. It can essentially improve treatment consistency and dynamic by creating valuable calculations. Artificial intelligence isn't just useful in the treatment of COVID-19–affected patients, but in addition to observing their legitimate wellbeing. It can follow the emergency of COVID-19 at various scales, for example, with clinical, atomic, and epidemiological applications. It is additionally useful to encourage the examination of this infection by breaking down the accessible information. Computer-based intelligence can help in creating legitimate treatment regimens, counteraction methodologies, medication, and immunization improvements (Ai et al., 2020).

8.4   CONCLUSION

The coronavirus pandemic has affected millions of people, leading to thousands of deaths globally. To contain the outbreak and continuous spread of the disease, countries imposed many regulations, such as quarantining people suspected of having contracted coronavirus, city lockdowns and the closure of borders, airport, and ports entries, businesses, sporting activities, and religious and social gatherings. The impact of these regulations has led to economic meltdown, loss of jobs, and hunger. Scientists from different fields have been in the warfront fighting against the virus via detection, treatment, and prevention. However, artificial intelligence-driven tools are part of the strong army that helps in predicting the spread of the viruses using regional or national datasets or datasets acquired from WHO, detecting infected people using chest X-ray scan images of patients with viral pneumonia, and identification of potential drugs based on simulations from available potent viral drugs against COVID-19.

8.5   FUTURE WORK

The COVID-19 pandemic stormed the world, which was not fully prepared, and that is why it spread faster and affected millions of people compared to other global pandemics, such as the Spanish flu, smallpox, Dengue virus, Ebola Virus, SARS, and MERS. The impact caused by this pandemic has now put scientists on alert, and will serve as motivation for the scientific community to intensify research on potential future outbreaks. The use of artificial intelligence has shown its efficiency as a system that can be use as either an alternative or confirmatory test for the detection of COVID-19, forecasting transmission and identification of potent drugs. However, the major limitations of this technique are acquiring more data which can help improve efficiency. Another challenge related to data acquisition is the privacy of medical data, which limits the use of artificial intelligence models to learn from vast amounts of data. Moreover, the integration of artificial intelligence and Internet of Things (IoT) is one of the possible tools that can help in detection, prediction, and the collection of data for data analysis for decision making. The system can also help in tracking disease all over the world, which will give scientists an opportunity to monitor, cure and prevent the spread of COVID-19.

REFERENCES

Ai, T., Z. Yang, H. Hou, C. Zhan, C. Chen, W. Lv et al. (2020). Correlation of chest CT and RT-PCR testing in coronavirus disease 2019 (COVID-19) in China: A report of 1014 cases. *Radiology*, 200642.

Apostolopoulos, I. D., & T. A. Mpesiana. (2020). Covid-19: Automatic detection from x-ray images utilizing transfer learning with convolutional neural networks. *Physical and Engineering Sciences in Medicine*, 1, 636–640.

Chan, J. F., K. H. Chan, R. Y. Kao, K. K. To, B. J. Zheng, C. P. Li et al. (2013). Broadspectrum antivirals for the emerging Middle East respiratory syndrome coronavirus. *Journal of Infection*, 67, 606–616.

Chan, J. F.-W., S. Yuan, K.-H. Kok, K. K.-W. To, H. Chu, J. Yang et al. (2020). A familial cluster of pneumonia associated with the 2019 novel coronavirus indicating person-to-person transmission: A study of a family cluster. *The Lancet*, 514–523.

Cui, J., F. Li, & Z. L. Shi. (2019). Origin and evolution of pathogenic coronaviruses. *Nature Reviews in Microbiology*, 17, 181–192.

Fan, Y., K. Zhao, Z. L. Shi, & P. Zhou. (2019). Bat coronaviruses in China. *Viruses*, 11(3), 210.

Gozes, O., M. Frid-Adar, H. Greenspan, P. D. Browning, H. Zhang, W. Ji et al. (2020). Rapid ai development cycle for the coronavirus (covid-19) pandemic: Initial results for automated detection & patient monitoring using deep learning ct image analysis. arXiv:2003.05037.

Haleem, A., M. Javaid, & I. H. Khan. (2019). Current status and applications of artificial intelligence (AI) in medical field: An overview. *Current Medicine Research and Practice*, 9(6), 231–237.

Hu, Z., Q. Ge, L. Jin, & M. Xiong. (2020). Artificial intelligence forecasting of covid-19 in China. arXiv:2002.07112.

Huang, C., Y. Wang, X. Li, L. Ren, J. Zhao, Y. Hu et al. (2020). Clinical features of patients infected with 2019 novel coronavirus in Wuhan, China. *The Lancet*, 395(10223), P497–506.

Jiang, X., M. Coffee, A. Bari, J. Wang, X. Jiang, J. Huang et al. (2020). Towards an artificial intelligence framework for data-driven prediction of coronavirus clinical severity. *CMC - Computers Materials & Continua*, 63(1), 537–551.

Kandeel, M., & M. Al-Nazawi. (2020). Virtual screening and repurposing of FDA approved drugs against COVID-19 main protease. *Life Sciences*, 251, 117627.

Khan, S., R. Siddique, M. A. Shereen, A. Ali, J. Liu, Q. Bai et al. (2020). Emergence of a novel coronavirus, severe acute respiratory syndrome coronavirus 2: Biology and therapeutic options. *Journal of Clinical Microbiology*, 58(5).

Kolhar, M., F. Al-Turjman, A. Alameen, M. Abualhaj, (2020). A three layered decentralized IoT biometric architecture for city lockdown during COVID-19 outbreak. *IEEE Access*, 8(1), 163608–163617.

Kumar, D., R. Malviya, & P. K. Sharma. (2020). Corona virus: A review of COVID-19. *Eurasian Journal of Medicine and Oncology*, 4, 8–25.

Letko M., & V. Munster. (2020). Functional assessment of cell entry and receptor usage for lineage B β-coronaviruses, including 2019nCoV. *bioRxiv*, 915660.

Long, J. B., & J. M. Ehrenfeld. (2020). The role of augmented intelligence (AI) in detecting and preventing the spread of novel coronavirus. *Journal of Medical Systems*, 44, 59.

Luo, H., Q. L. Tang, Y. X. Shang, S. B. Liang, M. Yang, N. Robinson, & J. P. Liu. (2020). Can Chinese medicine be used for prevention of corona virus disease 2019 (COVID-19)? A review of historical classics, research evidence and current prevention programs. *Chinese Journal of Integrative Medicine*, 26, 243–250.

Maghdid, H. S., K. Z. Ghafoor, A. S. Sadiq, K. Curran, & K. Rabie. (2020). A novel AI-enabled framework to diagnose coronavirus COVID 19 using smartphone embedded sensors: Design study. arXiv:2003.07434.

Miotto, R., F. Wang, S. Wang, X. Jiang, & J. T. Dudley. (2018). Deep learning for healthcare: Review, opportunities and challenges. *Briefings in Bioinformatics*, 19(6), 1236–1246.

Naylor, C. D. (2018). On the prospects for a (deep) learning health care system. *JAMA*, 320(11), 1099–1100.

Paules, C. I., H. D. Marston, & A. S. Fauci. (2020). Infeksi Coronavirus—Lebih dari Sekedar Pilek. *JAMA*, 323(8), 707–708.

Pirouz, B., S. Shaffiee Haghshenas, S. Shaffiee Haghshenas, & P. Piro. (2020). Investigating a serious challenge in the sustainable development process: Analysis of confirmed cases of COVID-19 (new type of coronavirus) through a binary classification using artificial intelligence and regression analysis. *Sustainability*, 12(6), 2427.

Sohrabi, C., Z. Alsafi, N. O'Neill, M. Khan, A. Kerwan, & A. Al-Jabir et al. (2020). Corrigendum to "World Health Organization declares Global Emergency: A review of the 2019 novel coronavirus (COVID-19)" [Int. J. Surg. 76 (2020) 71–76]. *International Journal of Surgery*, 77, 217. doi: 10.1016/j.ijsu.2020.03.036

Vaishya, R., M. Javaid, A. Haleem, I. Khan, & A. Vaish. (2020). Extending capabilities of artificial intelligence for decision-making and healthcare education. *Apollo Medicine*, 17, 53.

Waheed, A., M. Goyal, D. Gupta, A. Khanna, F. Al-Turjman, P. R. Pinheiro. (2020). CovidGAN: Data augmentation using auxiliary classifier GAN for improved Covid-19 detection, *IEEE Access*, 8, 91916–91923.

Wang, S., B. Kang, J. Ma, X. Zeng, M. Xiao, J. Guo, ... & B. Xu. (2020). A deep learning algorithm using CT images to screen for Corona Virus Disease (COVID-19). medRxiv. Published online April, 24, 2020–02.

Wynants, L., B. Van Calster, M. M. Bonten, G. S. Collins, T. P. Debray, M. De Vos et al. (2020). Prediction models for diagnosis and prognosis of covid-19 infection: Systematic review and critical appraisal. *bmj*, 369.

Xu, X., X. Jiang, C. Ma, P. Du, X. Li, S. Lv et al. (2020). Deep learning system to screen coronavirus disease 2019 pneumonia. arXiv:2002.09334.

Zeng, T., Y. Zhang, Z. Li, X. Liu, & B. Qiu. (2020). Predictions of 2019-nCoV transmission ending via comprehensive methods. arXiv:2002.04945.

Zhou, Y., Y. Hou, J. Shen, Y. Huang, W. Martin, & F. Cheng. (2020). Network-based drug repurposing for novel coronavirus 2019-nCoV/SARS-CoV-2. *Cell Discovery*, 6(1), 1–18.

Zu, Z. Y., M. D. Jiang, P. P. Xu, W. Chen, Q. Q. Ni, G. M. Lu, & L. J. Zhang. (2020). Coronavirus disease 2019 (COVID-19): A perspective from China. *Radiology*, 200490.

Zhao, Z., F. Zhang, M. Xu, K. Huang, W. Zhong, W. Cai, ... & J. Xiong. (2003). Description and clinical treatment of an early outbreak of severe acute respiratory syndrome (SARS) in Guangzhou, PR China. *Journal of Medical Microbiology*, 52(8), 715–720.

9 Physical Therapy Recommendations for Patients with COVID-19

Ayman A Mohamed, Motaz Alawna,
Fadi Al-Turjman, and Majdi Nassif

CONTENTS

9.1 INTRODUCTION

COVID-19 is a self-limited infection, in which the strength of the host's immune strength plays a significant role against it[1]. Thus, physical therapy could play an important role in increasing the immunity through increasing the aerobic capacity of these patients to improve their immune functions which would help counter COVID-19. Furthermore, pulmonary physical therapy could increase pulmonary functions, which could help in decreasing the COVID-19 associated pulmonary disorders and symptoms. This chapter discusses three main areas: (1) The effectiveness of increasing the aerobic capacity on immune and pulmonary functions, (2) The aerobic exercise recommendations for patients with COVID-19, and (3) The pulmonary exercises recommendations for patients with COVID-19.

9.1.1 LEARNING OBJECTIVES

After finishing reading this chapter, the readers will be able to:

- Know the importance of physical therapy for patients with COVID-19.
- Recognize the advantages of increasing the aerobic capacity on immune and pulmonary functions.

169

- Identify the aerobic exercises recommendations for patients with COVID-19.
- Identify the pulmonary exercises recommendations for patients with COVID-19.

9.2 THE EFFECT OF INCREASING THE AEROBIC CAPACITY ON IMMUNE AND PULMONARY FUNCTIONS

COVID-19 is considered a self-limited infection. In COVID-19, the immune strength plays a significant role to counter it[1]. Previously, it has been demonstrated that increasing the aerobic capacity causes short term effects on the immune system activity[2]. The effect of increasing the aerobic capacity on enhancing the immune functions mainly occurrs by three mechanisms. First, aerobic exercises elevate the function and level of immune cells in our bodies such as T-lymphocytes, macrophages, neutrophils, and monocytes; these cells are vital to counter any lung infections, including COVID-19[3–8]. Second, aerobic exercises raise the level and function of immunoglobulins (IgA, IgG, IgM,), principally IgA and IgM, because of their vital role against lung infections[9–12]. Third, aerobic exercises can adjust the level and function of C-reactive proteins (CRP) throughout, producing temporary small increases[13–15] to counter lung infections and, after a while, decreases to prevent its accompanying decrease in pulmonary functions[16, 17]. Aerobic exercises also lower the level of anxiety and depression, which helps to improve immune functions through different mechanisms, mainly by re-balancing T-helper-1/T-helper-2[18–24].

Increasing the aerobic capacity acts as a preventive and curable agent to counter respiratory infections and disorders. Increasing the aerobic capacity could prevent or decrease in the severity of both pneumonia[25–27] or acute respiratory distress syndrome (ARDS)[8,28,29]. These two disorders are mutual disorders in patients with COVID-19, and they are significantly responsible for the failure of the pulmonary system. Increasing the aerobic capacity improves lung functions and prevents lung damage through four main mechanisms. First, increasing the aerobic capacity acts as antimycotic prophylaxis and antibiotic to enhance lung and body immunity[27]. Second, increasing the aerobic capacity helps to restore normal lung tissue pliability and pulmonary muscle strength and endurance; this helps to enhance lung mechanics, ventilation, and lessenlung tissue damage[30–33]. Third, increasing the aerobic capacity acts as an antioxidant to decrease the accumulation of free radicals and oxidative destruction[34]. Fourth, increasing the aerobic capacity decreases the cough and clears respiratory airways throughout, enhancing the lung immunity[35] and modulating the autonomic system activity[36, 37]. Because of all these previous effects, increasing the aerobic capacity might have a more important role in pulmonary functions and immunity than usual breathing exercises, and can achieve additional improvements in cough mechanism[33, 38].

Furthermore, increasing the aerobic capacity can diminish COVID-19 risk factors. This helps in decreasing the incidence and progression of COVID-19. A recent study published on 13 March 2020[39] demonstrated that risk factors of COVID-19 increase the severity and death rates. These risk factors include aging, hypertension, diabetes, and heart problems. All these risk factors have been previously shown to be immediately or shortly improved by increasing the aerobic capacity[34, 40-46].

9.3 AEROBIC EXERCISE RECOMMENDATIONS FOR PATIENTS WITH COVID-19

Generally, a routine of mild-to-moderate aerobic exercises performed for 10–30 min should be followed by all people in lockdown or patients with mild pulmonary symptoms. Several studies demonstrated the short-term effects of performing mild-to-moderate aerobic exercises on enhancing both immune and pulmonary functions.

Concerning the effect of increasing the aerobic capacity on immune functions, several studies have demonstrated the short-term effects of aerobic exercises on enhancing immune functions. Gonçalves et al.[3] reported that aerobic exercises produce fast and short-term enhancements in the level and function of T-lymphocytes, leukocytes, subpopulations, immunoglobulins, and interleukins. Lippi et al.[4, 5] have shown that mild aerobic exercises increase the level of monocyte, neutrophil, and leukocyte. Lira et al.[7] have demonstrated that in the 60 minutes following a 5km run, an increase in cytokine IL-6 and IL-10 occurs. Li et al.[6] have reported that one session of prolonged mild aerobic exercises elevates the amount of blood neutrophil, leukocyte, and monocyte for up to nine hours.

Concerning the effect of increasing aerobic capacity on pulmonary functions, several studies have demonstrated the short-term effects of aerobic exercises on enhancing pulmonary functions in either pneumonia or ARDS. Williams[47] has demonstrated that mild aerobic exercise, like running and walking, decreases the risk of respiratory diseases and pneumonia. Neuman et al.[25] have reported that aerobic exercises reduce the incidence of pneumonia in women in the US. Olivo et al.[26] have demonstrated that mild aerobic exercises have an anti-inflammatory effect, decreasing lung inflammation present in patients with streptococcus pneumonia. Vieira et al.[48] have demonstrated that increasing the aerobic capacity increases levels of immune cells, particularly, IL-10, which has a vital role in immunity to counter acute lung inflammations and injuries. A very recent study conducted by Shi et al.[29] demonstrated that five weeks of mild aerobic exercises can prevent acute lung injury in mice.

Furthermore, increasing aerobic exercises can decrease risk factors of COVID-19, which could help in decreasing its incidence or severity. Yokoyama et al.[42] have shown that mild aerobic exercises performed for 45 minutes for thee weeks significantly decreased arterial stiffness in both common carotid and femoral arteries, and this decrease was accompanied by an augmentation in insulin resistance. Charlotte et al.[49] have reported that one session of aerobic exercises significantly decreases the ambulatory BP up to 25 hours after the session. Guimaraes et al.[50] have demonstrated that two weeks of mild aerobic exercises significantly lowers both diastolic and systolic BP and cardiovascular load after the exercise, and this decrease continues up to 24 hours after the session in patients with resistant hypertension. Cahapman et al.[43] have demonstrated that mild aerobic exercises performed for six weeks significantly elevated both VO_2 max and perceived exertion rate. Francesco et al.[44] have shown that mild aerobic exercises performed for eight weeks significantly raised VO_2 peak uptake, heart rate recovery, and ventilatory and aerobic thresholds, and decreased the rate of the rise of ventilation/unit of carbon dioxide production.

9.4 PULMONARY EXERCISES RECOMMENDATIONS FOR PATIENTS WITH COVID-19

Pulmonary exercises should be an essential element in the treatment of patients with COVID-19 because of COVID-19 targets mainly the pulmonary system. Pneumonia and ARDS are the two main disorders leading to death in patients with COVID-19. Also, pulmonary exercises can decrease coughing, which is considered one of the main signs and symptoms of COVID-19.

Pulmonary exercises have been demonstrated to increase lung functions, elasticity, and strength; these are very important in helping patients with COVID-19 to recover faster and decreasing the death rate. Vieira et al.[51] have reported that breathing exercises significantly improve all breathing patterns and thoracoabdominal motions. Lee et al.[52] have shown that one session of respiratory exercises significantly enhances the forced expiratory volume and forced vital capacity in one second.

Pulmonary exercises significantly decrease the signs and symptoms of pneumonia. It has been demonstrated that deep breathing exercises can be utilized to reduce the prevalence and severity of pulmonary complications, such as atelectasis, pneumonia, and hypoxemia[53,54]. Liu et al.[55] have demonstrated that pulmonary rehabilitation significantly decreases pneumonia severity and increases the pulmonary functions in patients with severe pneumonia. Chigira et al.[56] has reported that early pulmonary exercises, consisting of breathing exercises and postural drainage, significantly decrease the severity and complications of pneumonia and enhance lung functions.

Also, pulmonary exercises significantly decrease the signs and symptoms of ARDS. Gai et al.[57] have reported that a pulmonary exercise program, consisting of percussion on back, roll over, postural drainage, and manipulative lung inflation, significantly increases all oxygen parameters (PaO_2, $PaCO_2$, $PaO2/FiO_2$) and decreases the lung complications in patients with respiratory failure. Haren et al.[58] have shown that breathing exercises using mechanical ventilation decrease the severity and complications of ARDS. Putensen et al.[59] have revealed that assisted breathing exercises significantly improve pulmonary gas exchange, systemic blood flow, and oxygen supply to the tissue in patients with acute respiratory failure.

There are different types of pulmonary exercises that help in decreasing both moist or dry coughs. One of the most-used pulmonary exercises used to get rid of sputum, and that consequently improves the lung function, is postural drainage[60]. Percussion is another pulmonary technique that could be used to get rid of sputum and improve lung function[61]. Also, there are various pulmonary exercises that can be used to enhance the dry cough commonly seen in patients with COVID-19.

As mentioned earlier, aerobic exercises improve the dry cough more than breathing exercises[36, 37], because aerobic exercise causes autonomic modulation, which helps significantly in decreasing the bronchospasm mainly responsible for dry cough[62].

REFERENCES

1. Cascella, M,. M. Rajnik, A. Cuomo, S. C. Dulebohn, and R. Di Napoli. (2020). *Features, Evaluation and Treatment Coronavirus (COVID-19)*.
2. Mohamed, A., and M. Alawna. (2020). Role of increasing the aerobic capacity on improving the function of immune and respiratory systems in patients with coronavirus (COVID-19): A review. *Diabetes & Metabolic Syndrome: Clinical Research & Reviews*, 14(4): 489–496.
3. Gonçalves, C. A. M., P. M. S. Dantas, I. K. dos Santos et al. (2020). Effect of acute and chronic aerobic exercise on immunological markers: A systematic review. *Frontiers in Physiology*, , 10(January): 1–11.
4. Lippi, G., G. Banfi, M. Montagnana, G. L. Salvagno, F. Schena, and G. C. Guidi. (2010). Acute variation of leucocytes counts following a half-marathon run. *International Journal of Laboratory Hematology*, 32(1 PART.2): 117–121.
5. Lippi, G., G. L. Salvagno, E. Danese et al. (2014). Mean platelet volume (MPV) predicts middle distance running performance. *PLoS One*, 9(11): 8–13.
6. Li, T. L., and P. Y. Cheng. (2007). Alterations of immunoendocrine responses during the recovery period after acute prolonged cycling. *European Journal of Applied Physiology*, 101(5): 539–546.
7. Lira, F. S., T. dos Santos, R. S. Caldeira et al. (2017). Short-term high- and moderate-intensity training modifies inflammatory and metabolic factors in response to acute exercise. *Frontiers in Physiology*, 8(OCT): 1–8.
8. Reis Gonçalves, C. T., C. G. Reis Gonçalves, F. M. de Almeida et al. (2012). Protective effects of aerobic exercise on acute lung injury induced by LPS in mice. *Critical Care*, 16(5): R199.
9. Rodríguez, A., A. Tjärnlund, J. Ivanji et al. (2005). Role of IgA in the defense against respiratory infections: IgA deficient mice exhibited increased susceptibility to intranasal infection with Mycobacterium bovis BCG. *Vaccine*, 23(20): 2565–2572.
10. Hines, M. T., H. C. Schott, W. M. Bayly, and A. J. Leroux. (1996). Exercise and immunity: A review with emphasis on the horse. *Journal of Veterinary Internal Medicine*, 10(10): 280–289.
11. Cunningham-Rundles, C. (2009). Lung disease, antibodies and other unresolved issues in immune globulin therapy for antibody deficiency. *Clinical and Experimental Immunology*, 157 Supplement 1: 12–16.
12. Mohamed, G., and M. Taha. (2016). Comparison between the effects of aerobic and resistive training on immunoglobulins in obese women. *Bulletin of Faculty of Physical Therapy*, 21(1): 11.
13. Pedersen, B. K., and L. Hoffman-Goetz. (2000). Exercise and the immune system: Regulation, integration, and adaptation. *Physiological Reviews*, 80(3): 1055–1081.
14. Marklund, P., C. M. Mattsson, B. Wåhlin-Larsson et al. Extensive inflammatory cell infiltration in human skeletal muscle in response to an ultraendurance exercise bout in experienced athletes. *Journal of Applied Physiology*, 114(1): 66–72.
15. De Gonzalo-Calvo, D., A. Dávalos, A. Montero et al. (2015). Circulating inflammatory miRNA signature in response to different doses of aerobic exercise. *Journal of Applied Physiology*, 119(2): 124–134.

16. Zheng, G., P. Qiu, R. Xia et al. (2019). Effect of aerobic exercise on inflammatory markers in healthy middle-aged and older adults: A systematic review and meta-analysis of randomized controlled trials. *Frontiers in Aging Neuroscience*, 11(Apr): 98.

17. Okita, K., H. Nishijima, T. Murakami et al. (2004). Can exercise training with weight loss lower serum C-reactive protein levels? *Arteriosclerosis, thrombosis, and vascular biology*, 24(10): 1868–1873.

18. Marshall, G. D. (2011). The adverse effects of psychological stress on immunoregulatory balance: Applications to human inflammatory diseases. *Immunology and Allergy Clinics,* 31(1): 133–140.

19. Reed, J., and S. Buck. (2009). The effect of regular aerobic exercise on positive-activated affect: A meta-analysis. *Psychology of Sport and Exercise*, 10(6): 581–594.

20. Chan, J. S. Y., G. Liu, D. Liang, K. Deng, J. Wu, and J. H. Yan. (2019). Special issue–therapeutic benefits of physical activity for mood: A systematic review on the effects of exercise intensity, duration, and modality. *Journal of Psychology*, 153(1): 102–125.

21. Hogan, C. L., J. Mata, and L. L. Carstensen. (2013). Exercise holds immediate benefits for affect and cognition in younger and older adults. *Psychology and Aging*, 28(2): 587–594.

22. Broman-Fulks, J. J., and K. M. Storey. (2008). Evaluation of a brief aerobic exercise intervention for high anxiety sensitivity. *Anxiety, Stress & Coping*, 21(2): 117–128.

23. Crabbe, J. B., J. C. Smith, and R. K. Dishman. (2007). Emotional & electroencephalographic responses during affective picture viewing after exercise ☆. *Physiology and Behavior*, 90: 394–404.

24. Nabkasorn, C., N. Miyai, A. Sootmongkol et al. (2006). Effects of physical exercise on depression, neuroendocrine stress hormones and physiological fitness in adolescent females with depressive symptoms. *European Journal of Public Health*, 16(2): 179–184.

25. Neuman, M. I., W. C. Willett, and G. C. Curhan. (2010). Physical activity and the risk of community-acquired pneumonia in US women. *American Journal of Medicine*, 123(3): 1–10.

26. Olivo, C. R., E. N. Miyaji, M. L. S. Oliveira et al. (2014). Aerobic exercise attenuates pulmonary inflammation induced by Streptococcus pneumoniae. *Journal of Applied Physiology*, 117(9): 998–1007.

27. Baumann, F. T., P. Zimmer, K. Finkenberg, M. Hallek, W. Bloch, and T. Elter. (2012). Influence of endurance exercise on the risk of pneumonia and fever in leukemia and lymphoma patients undergoing high dose chemotherapy. A pilot study. *Journal of Sports Science & Medicine*, 11(4): 638–642.

28. Rigonato-Oliveira, N. C., B. A. Mackenzie, A. L. L. Bachi et al. (2018). Aerobic exercise inhibits acute lung injury: From mouse to human evidence exercise reduced lung injury markers in mouse and in cells. *Exercise Immunology Review*, 24: 36–44.

29. Shi, Y., T. Liu, D. C. Nieman et al. Aerobic exercise attenuates acute lung injury through NET inhibition. *Frontiers in Immunology*, 11: 409.

30. Toledo, A. C., R. M. Magalhaes, D. C. Hizume et al. (2012). Aerobic exercise attenuates pulmonary injury induced by exposure to cigarette smoke. *European Respiratory Journal*, 39(2): 254–264.

31. Guimarães, I., G. Padilha, M. Lopes-Pacheco et al. (2011). The impact of aerobic exercise on lung inflammation and remodeling in experimental emphysema. *European Respiratory Journal*, 38:4733.

32. Dassios, T., A. Katelari, S. Doudounakis, and G. Dimitriou. (2013). Aerobic exercise and respiratory muscle strength in patients with cystic fibrosis. *Respiratory Medicine*, 107(5): 684––690.

33. Yamashina, Y, H. Aoyama, H. Hori et al. (2019). Comparison of respiratory muscle strength in individuals performing continuous and noncontinuous walking exercises in water after the 6-week program. *Journal of exercise rehabilitation*, 15(4): 566–570.

34. Stravinskas Durigon, T., B. A. Mackenzie, M. Carneiro Oliveira-Junior et al. (2018). Aerobic exercise protects from pseudomonas aeruginosa -induced pneumonia in elderly mice. *Journal of Innate Immunity*, 10(4): 279–290.

35. Vieira, R. P., A. C. de Toledo, S. C. Ferreira et al. (2011). Airway epithelium mediates the anti-inflammatory effects of exercise on asthma. *Respiratory Physiology and Neurobiology*, 175(3): 383–389.

36. Leite, M. R., E. M. C. Ramos, C. A. Kalva-Filho et al. (2015). Effects of 12 weeks of aerobic training on autonomic modulation, mucociliary clearance, and aerobic parameters in patients with COPD. *International Journal of Chronic Obstructive Pulmonary Disease*, 10(1): 2549–2557.

37. Borghi-Silva, A., R. Arena, V. Castello et al. (2009). Aerobic exercise training improves autonomic nervous control in patients with COPD. *Respiratory Medicine*, 103(10): 1503–1510.

38. Evaristo, K. B., M. G. Saccomani, M. A. Martins et al. (2014). Comparison between breathing and aerobic exercise on clinical control in patients with moderate-to-severe asthma: Protocol of a randomized trial. *BMC Pulmonary Medicine*, 14: 160.

39. Wu, C., X. Chen, Y. Cai et al. (2020). Risk factors associated with acute respiratory distress syndrome and death in patients with coronavirus disease 2019 pneumonia in Wuhan, China. *JAMA Internal Medicine*, 180(7): 1–10.

40. Bacchi, E., C. Negri, M. Trombetta et al. (2012). Differences in the acute effects of aerobic and resistance exercise in subjects with type 2 diabetes: Results from the RAED2 randomized trial. *PLoS One*, 7(12): e49937.

41. Yardley, J. E., G. P. Kenny, B. A. Perkins et al. (2013). Resistance versus aerobic exercise. *Diabetes Care*, 36(3): 537–542.

42. Yokoyama, H., M. Emoto, S. Fujiwara et al. (2004). Short-term aerobic exercise improves arterial stiffness in type 2 diabetes. *Diabetes Research and Clinical Practice*, 65(2): 85–93.

43. Chapman, S. B., S. Aslan, J. S. Spence et al. (2013). Shorter term aerobic exercise improves brain, cognition, and cardiovascular fitness in aging. *Frontiers in Aging Neuroscience*, 5: 75.

44. Giallauria, F., D. Del Forno, F. Pilerci et al. (2005). Improvement of heart rate recovery after exercise training in older people. *Journal of the American Geriatrics Society*, 53(11), 2037–2038.

45. Tao, L., Y. Bei, S. Lin et al. (2015). Exercise training protects against acute myocardial infarction via improving myocardial energy metabolism and mitochondrial biogenesis. *Cellular Physiology and Biochemistry*, 37(1): 162–175.

46. Wisløff, U., J. P. Loennechen, S. Currie, G. L. Smith, and Ø, Ellingsen. (2002). Aerobic exercise reduces cardiomyocyte hypertrophy and increases contractility, Ca2+ sensitivity and SERCA-2 in rat after myocardial infarction. *Cardiovascular Research*, 54(1): 162–174.

47. Williams, P. T. (2014). Dose-response relationship between exercise and respiratory disease mortality. *Medicine and Science in Sports and Exercise*, 46(4):711–717.

48. Vieira, R. P., M. C. Oliveira-Junior, R. W. Teixeira et al. (2013). The crucial role of IL-10 in the anti-inflammatory effects of aerobic exercise in a model LPS-induced ARDS. *European Respiratory Journal*, 42: 4402.

49. Lund Rasmussen, C., L. Nielsen, M. Linander Henriksen et al. (2018). Acute effect on ambulatory blood pressure from aerobic exercise: a randomised cross-over study among female cleaners. *European Journal of Applied Physiology*, 118(2): 331–338.

50. Guimarães, G. V., L. G. B. Cruz, A. C. Tavares, E. L. Dorea, M. M. Fernandes-Silva, and E. A. Bocchi. (2013). Effects of short-term heated water-based exercise training on systemic blood pressure in patients with resistant hypertension. *Blood Pressure Monitoring*18, 342–345.

51. Vieira, D. S. R., L. P. S. Mendes, N. S. Elmiro, M. Velloso, R. R. Britto, and V. F. Parreira. (2014). Breathing exercises: Influence on breathing patterns and thoracoabdominal motion in healthy subjects. *Brazilian Journal of Physical Therapy*, 18(6): 544–552.

52. Lee, D.-K., H.-J. Jeong, and J.-S. Lee. (2018). Effect of respiratory exercise on pulmonary function, balance, and gait in patients with chronic stroke. *Journal of Physical Therapy Science*, 30(8): 984–987.

53. Hinkle, J. L., and K. H. Cheever. (2010). Preoperative nursing management. In *Brunner and Suddarth's Textbook of Medical-Surgical*, Smeltzer, S. C., Bare, B. G., Hinkle, J. L. and K. H. Cheever (Eds.), 12th ed. (425–441). Philadelphia, PA: Lippincott Williams & Wilkins.

54. Ünver, S., G. Kıvanç, and H. M. Alptekin. (2018). Deep breathing exercise education receiving and performing status of patients undergoing abdominal surgery. *International Journal of Health Sciences (Qassim)*, 12(4): 35–38.

55. Liu, W., X. Mu, X. Wang, P. Zhang, L. Zhao, and Q. Li. (2018). Effects of comprehensive pulmonary rehabilitation therapy on pulmonary functions and blood gas indexes of patients with severe pneumonia. *Experimental and Therapeutic Medicine*, 16(3): 1953–1957.

56. Chigira, Y., T. Takai, H. Igusa, and K. Dobashi. (2015). Effects of early physiotherapy with respect to severity of pneumonia of elderly patients admitted to an intensive care unit: A single center study in Japan. *Journal of Physical Therapy Science*, 27(7): 2053–2056.

57. Gai, L., Y. Tong, and B. Yan. (2018). The effects of pulmonary physical therapy on the patients with respiratory failure. *Iranian Journal of Public Health*, 47(7): 1001–1006.

58. Van Haren, F., T. Pham, L. Brochard et al. (2019). Spontaneous breathing in early acute respiratory distress syndrome: Insights from the large observational study to understand the global impact of severe acute respiratory failure study∗. *Critical Care Medicine*, 47(2): 229–238.

59. Putensen, C., R. Hering, T. Muders, and H. Wrigge. (2005). Assisted breathing is better in acute respiratory failure. *Current Opinion in Critical Care*, 11(1): 63–68.

60. Ntoumenopoulos, G., A. Gild, and D. J. Cooper. (1998). The effect of manual lung hyperinflation and postural drainage on pulmonary complications in mechanically ventilated trauma patients. *Anaesthesia and Intensive Care*, 26(5): 492–496.

61. Varekojis, S. M., F. H. Douce, R. L. Flucke et al. (2003). A comparison of the therapeutic effectiveness of and preference for postural drainage and percussion, intrapulmonary percussive ventilation, and high-frequency chest wall compression in hospitalized cystic fibrosis patients. *Respiratory Care*, 48(1): 24–28.

62. Overlack, A. (1996). ACE inhibitor-induced cough and bronchospasm. Incidence, mechanisms and management. *Drug Safety*, 15(1): 72–78.

10 AI in Fighting against COVID-19

A Case Study

Deepanshu Srivastava, S. Rakeshkumar,
N. Gayathri, and Fadi Al-Turjman

CONTENTS

10.1   INTRODUCTION

COVID-19 (2019 novel coronavirus) is a viral respiratory illness caused by a coronavirus that has not been found in people before. It can lead to lower respiratory illnesses like pneumonia and bronchitis. The coronavirus has put almost the entire world on high alert, with cases of infection having been reported on every continent except for Antarctica. We can only hope that India does not become one of its permanent hotspots.

The preventive measures are taken by the government and various medical institutions. As responsible citizens of our country, it is the duty of each one of us to take care that the infection, as well as fake information, does not spread.

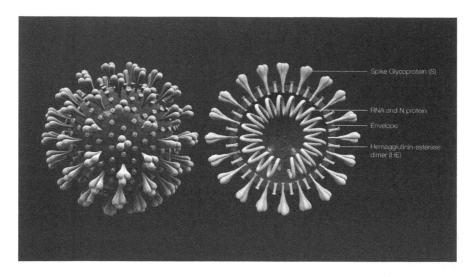

FIGURE 10.1   Structure of coronavirus.

COVID-19 is spread through respiratory droplets of infected individuals from coughing, sneezing, etc.; close contact with an infected person (within 6 feet); and possibly through contact with infected surfaces or objects, then touching of the mouth, nose, or eyes. Carelessness by any of us can lead to a serious outcome for the society, city, state, and then to whole country [1, 2] (Figure 10.1).

10.2   SYMPTOMS

1. Fever, cough, and shortness of breath.
2. Symptoms may appear 2–14 days after exposure.

10.3   PREVENTION

Prevention guidelines provided by top the medical department (World Health Organization [WHO]) are:

1. When an individual has come from outside, avoid touching the eyes, nose, and mouth.
2. Regularly clean your hands with an alcohol-based hand rub or wash them with soap.
3. If you feel unwell, then don't go to work, and immediately report to the nearest hospital.
4. Maintain social distancing.
5. It takes between 5 and 10 days before people who are infected become corona-positive, so major care is to be taken during these days.

At the time of writing, the six countries in the high-risk categories are: China, Iran, South Korea, Japan, Italy, and Mongolia. If you have travelled overseas to countries

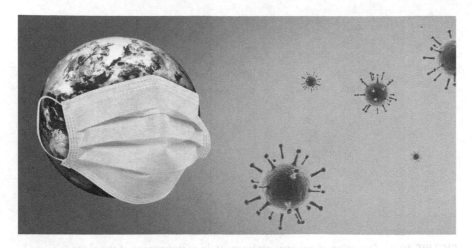

FIGURE 10.2 Figure depicting the necessity of a safe environment to fight against coronavirus.

where there is a travel advisory of "do not travel," "reconsider the need to travel," or "exercise a high degree of caution," or if you have had contact with a person who has travelled to such a country, we respectfully request that travelers returning from these countries follow government-enforced quarantine protocols; practice good hygiene, including hand washing or applying alcohol-based sanitizer before entering the country.

Avoid touching all fixtures, fittings, and furniture within the home, and instead, ask our agents to demonstrate the functionality of any devices if required [2, 10] (Figure 10.2).

10.4   PREPARATION FOR COVID-19

1. Establish communication with your local health department to stay informed about COVID-19.
2. Know how and where to report and refer potential cases for testing; identify COVID-19 testing locations.
3. Establish, review, and update your emergency plan.
4. Collect sanitation supplies as available – masks, alcohol-based sanitizer, cleaning supplies, linens.
5. Identify isolation spaces for sick individuals.
6. Be aware of school/business closures – they may impact staff, volunteers, and clients [2] (Figures 10.3 & 10.4).

10.5   TESTING FOR COVID-19

1. If the client has severe symptoms (extreme difficulty breathing, bluish lips or face, etc.), call and notify your public health department.
2. Limit the number of staff entering and exiting the room, and document staff that have had contact with sick clients.

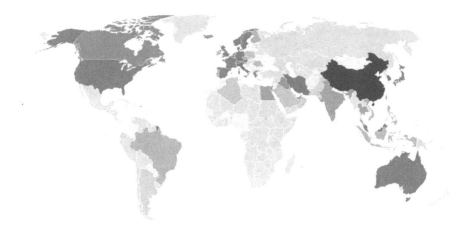

FIGURE 10.3   Depiction of coronavirus intensity in various areas of the globe.

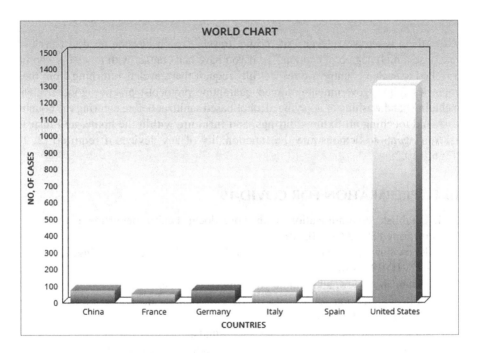

FIGURE 10.4   World chart (major countries affected with corona).

3. Staff should wear facemasks, gloves, gowns, and eye protection when engaging sick clients, and wash hands thoroughly before and afterwards.
4. Sick clients should be encouraged not to interact with pets. If they do, encourage harm-reduction strategies, such as frequent hand washing and not sleeping with pets [2, 10] (Figure 10.5).

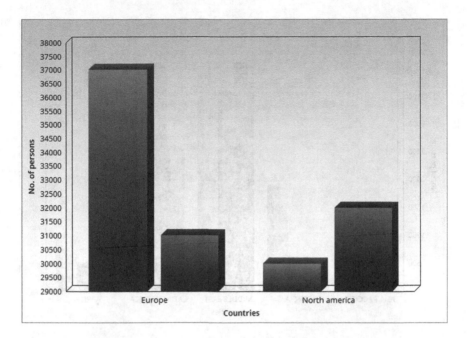

FIGURE 10.5 Position of Europe and North American countries condition during coronavirus.

10.6 FORMATION OF VIRUSES

Human viruses cannot grow in foods. Since viruses are very host-specific, a human virus will rarely multiply in food, even in foods that are still alive (like oysters). However, they can persist for a long time.

The cell walls of plants are tough, and plant viruses have no specific mechanism for entering the host cell. Person-to-person transmission is the way it is spreading, as shown by significant growth in the various or mostly all countries.

The novel coronavirus was first identified in Wuhan in China. According to research and various studies, a woman travelled from Wuhan to another part of China called Anyang in January. There, she met with people as well as patients [3] (Figure 10.6).

Initially, no cases or reports were found at the hospital or other campuses, since the patients were isolated. Later, in the month of February, she found bad health conditions were affecting areas of the chest and throat, followed by fever [3].

European food safety authority (EFSA) is closely monitoring the situation regarding the outbreak of COVID-19 that is affecting a large number of countries across the globe. There is currently no evidence that food is a likely source or route of transmission of the virus.

EFSA's chief scientist, Marta Hugas, said: "Experiences from previous outbreaks of related coronaviruses, such as severe acute respiratory syndrome coronavirus (SARS—CoV) [and]

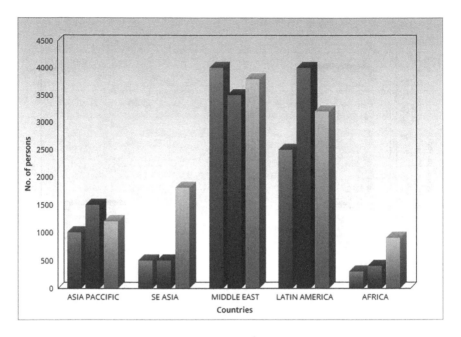

FIGURE 10.6   Position of Big Giants Countries' conditions during coronavirus spread.

Middle East respiratory syndrome coronavirus (MERS—CoV), show that transmission through food consumption did not occur. At the moment, there is no evidence to suggest that coronavirus is any different in this respect [3]."

10.7   PREVENTION OF VIRUSES THROUGH ANTIOXIDANTS

Vitamin C serves essential roles in the human body and supports normal immune function. As an antioxidant, the vitamin neutralizes charged particles, called free radicals, that can damage tissues in the body.

It also helps the body synthesize hormones, build collagen, and seal off vulnerable connective tissue against pathogens. So yes, vitamin C should absolutely be included in your daily diet if you want to maintain a healthy immune system [4, 9] (Figure 10.7).

However, mega dosing on supplements is unlikely to lower your risk of catching COVID-19, and may, at most give you a "modest" advantage against the virus, should you become infected.

No evidence suggests that other so-called immune-boosting supplements – such as zinc, green tea, or Echinacea – help to prevent COVID-19, either [4].

10.8   HERBS AS ANTIOXIDANTS

The herb Echinacea (*Echinacea purpurea*) is supportive of the immune system and has a direct anti-viral action against colds and viral bronchitis. Preparations that

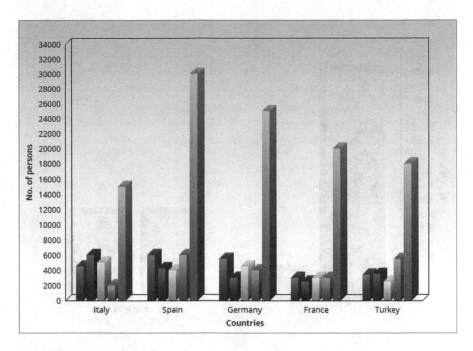

FIGURE 10.7 Conditions of Italy, Spain, Germany, France, turkey, UK, and the US.

include both the roots and the flowering tops are the most effective at helping the body resist the viruses.

If we are able to spread this all over the world, it may be possible to kill the coronavirus in the air, or antiviral medicine powder can help us to do so, and measures that are hygienic can work to reduce the rate of transmission [5] (Figure 10.8).

The cold caused by the coronavirus can be diagnosed clinically, as it is different from the cold of an individual. On the basis of antibody tests in paired sera, the laboratory is trying their best to give provide a solution as early as possible because Isolation is difficult for this virus, these nucleic acid hybridization tests with PCR [6, 8] (Figure 10.9).

10.9 LONG-TERM IMPLICATIONS

Due to this severe situation, some people are also creating fake opportunity scams, so that they can take someone's hard-earned money. In recent months, several students have been the victims of online job opportunity scams. The scammers make contact via email with a job offer.

After accepting the offer, the victim is sent checks to deposit with instructions to return a portion of the money to the scammer using a money transfer app. Soon after, funds are stolen from the victim's account by the scammer. Be advised that this scam is still occurring, now under the guise of working at home due to the COVID-19 outbreak. Legitimate employment and job offers are not handled this way.

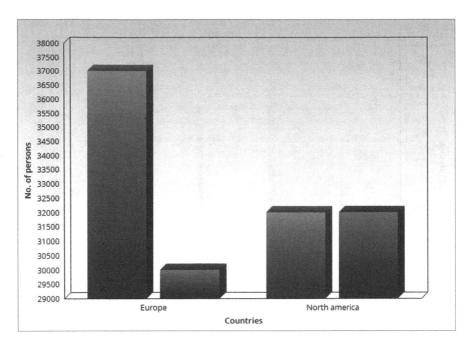

FIGURE 10.8   Condition of Europe and North America – rise in no. of cases over a period of time.

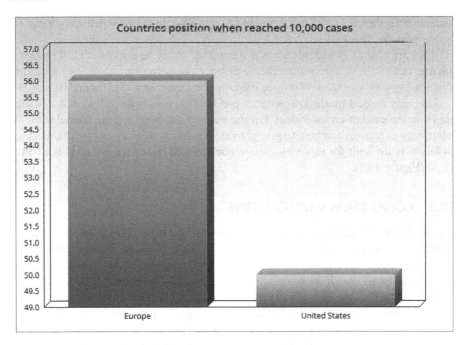

FIGURE 10.9   Position of Europe and US conditions when they reached 10,000 cases.

As always, one should be extremely cautious about interacting with someone they don't know, especially online. Never provide access to sensitive personal information.

1. Downward pressure on the on-demand economy and a reversion towards asset ownership and control.
2. Increase in desirability of full-time work vs. participating in on-demand jobs and marketplaces.
3. Broad flight towards job-security with the best, most profitable companies.
4. Broad exacerbation of inequality issues and social challenges.
5. Reorganization of government tactics for supporting people during a shock.
6. Move towards strong national ID.
7. Acceptance of increased state surveillance and border hardening.
8. Pressure towards digital voting, remote services, and Drone iBot delivery.
9. Pressure to decentralize production facilities, knowledge, work, and education.
10. Possible decline in cities and commercial real estate.
11. Adoption of VR, Peloton, etc.
12. Shifts in event businesses.
13. Shifts in trust [6, 8].

10.10 CASE STUDY OF FISH WORKER COMMUNITY

Due to these severe conditions, the small worker sector is highly affected by COVID-19. This includes the fish worker community, a community with a major number of migrants to other occupations and areas.

As such, this community should be very vigilant about its members coming home from outside and possible contraction of infection. All the general instructions for protection, including lock down, should be translated into the specific community situation, and have to be strictly followed.

They should practice the following:

Marine fishing requires collective activity. Each fisher team should ensure that none of their members have any related symptom before coming together to go for fishing

Fishing crews in larger boats going for multi-day fishing should ensure that no fish worker with related symptoms boards the boat. Multi-day fishing should be avoided as much as possible.

All fish landing centers and fishing harbors should ensure thermal screening of fish workers boarding on and alighting from fishing vessels with follow-up measures. Masks should be kept on board for use of any crew member who may show symptoms while on the fishing voyage.

Immediate voluntary quarantine and follow-up testing with treatment should be resorted to in the event of any fish worker showing symptoms of coronavirus sickness on or off work. While transporting the fish, masks should be used, with adequate hand washing before and after transportation [11] (Figure 10.10).

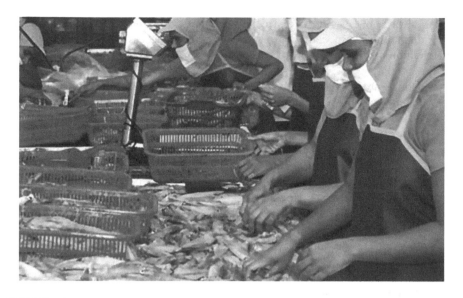

FIGURE 10.10   Workers using masks and suits to prevent the coronavirus.

Many fish vendors or fish sorters and dryers come together to transact and work on the beach. They should have masks and wash their hands as often as possible. Avoid touching the face or nose.

Auction centers, either on the beach or at designated places, are the next points of mass contact. The fishers and fish vendors, marine or inland, who attend the auction centers for selling and buying fish, must use masks and have facilities for recurrent and adequate hand washing with soap and water.

Avoid touching the face or nose. Fish vendors should use masks and have soap and water for recurrent and adequate hand washing.

The civil administration should be requested to ensure –

Easy and prompt access to medical advice, testing and treatment (essential in lockdown period); adequate supply of rations with cooking fuel to the small-scale fish workers; monetary allowance to attend to other essential needs during lockdown and the affected period;

supply of masks with proper instructions on its use and use of soap and water; and awareness building campaigns in fishing community hubs in collaboration with local fish worker organizations [11].

10.11   ARTIFICIAL INTELLIGENCE (AI) AND MACHINE LEARNING (ML) IN COVID-19 [12, 13]

Data Science can save lives today. AI and ML are incredible forces to do good for humanity. The problems that can be solved through AI and ML techniques are:

1. Hospital staffing predictions.
2. ICU transfers and triage.

3. Population risk segmentation.
4. Predicting the spread of COVID-19.
5. Predicting operational efficiency and resilience during a pandemic.
6. Hospital supply chain predictions.
7. Predicting responses by city, hospitals, and Sepsis predictions (Figure 10.11).
   - Data sets: H2O.ai is evaluating global and open health data sets to determine patterns.
   - Expertise: H2O.ai's data science experts are contributing their knowledge to solve pressing problems with the pandemic.
   - AI platforms: H2O.ai is contributing its Driverless AI and Q platform to model, predict, and visualize data sets.
   - AI solutions: H2O.ai is creating pandemic- and health-specific solutions for general use.

AI is making waves in healthcare, with its immense potential to analyze complex data and extract meaningful insights in order to improve the entire patient journey, which includes different aspects of patient care along with other processes.

Organizations like care-providers, payers, pharmaceuticals, and the life sciences have already employed AI in the areas of diagnosis and treatment (prediction to improve diagnoses, disease classification, etc.), patient engagement, recommendation, and other administrative activities.

Research says that 40 per cent of the tasks performed by clinical staff and 33 per cent of the clinical jobs can be managed by AI, machine learning, and RPA solution through automation. Other areas where AI is being leveraged is for automating the repetitive and complex tasks which primarily depended on human inputs, for example, radiologists for spotting malignant tumors, or other workflows like revenue cycle management, patient appointment scheduling, billing and account settlement, insurance claims, supply chain, and inventory management.

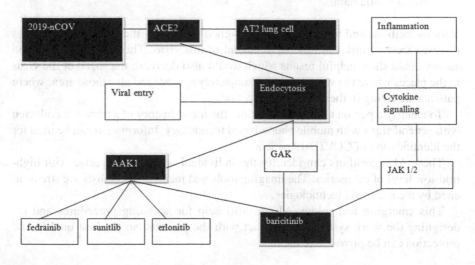

FIGURE 10.11   COVID-19 with machine learning.

Basically, it will transform the way patient care and administrative tasks can be managed, resulting in reduced medical staff burnout, better interoperability, and growth in revenues. With automation, healthcare professionals can now utilize and leverage their skills in more valuable tasks.

AI can also be useful in the area of a general medical situation, where a lot of repeating tests are conducted for similar symptoms of diseases, which in turn will save time and increase the accuracy of the findings.

Hospitals will gain lots of advantages and potential by improving the way patients are treated, including the time of stay or correct combination of medicines, etc. AI-driven smart insights can build their capabilities even further.

10.12   ARTIFICIAL INTELLIGENCE (AI) ALGORITHMS

AI Algorithm Parameters:

1. **Detection**: early warning; detecting anomalies and digital "smoke signals," like BlueDot.
   Diagnosis: pattern recognition using medical imagery and symptom data.
2. **Prevention**: prediction; calculating a person's probability of infection.
   Surveillance: to monitor and track contagion in real time, e.g. contact tracing.
   Information: personalized news and content moderation to fight misinformation, e.g. via social networks.
3. **Response**: delivery drones for materials transport; robots for high-exposure tasks at hospitals, e.g. CRUZR robot.
   Service automation: deploying triaging virtual assistants and chatbots, like Canada's COVID-19 chatbot.
4. **Recovery**: monitor; track economic recovery through satellite, GPS, and social media data.

Various methods and techniques were designed to identify the COVID-19 virus, as this was the first task towards the treatment of this virus. The mobile phone-based survey could show helpful results which would also decrease the speed of the virus in the places where the virus has been completely spread, and also those areas where patients are living in their quarantine sections.

To identify a person under investigation, the travel history of a person is collected with general signs with mobile phone-based technology. Information can be used for the identification of COVID-19 patients.

These AI algorithms can identify the individual and can categorize with high-mid-low level of categories. The imaging tools and medical specialists are strengthened by the use of AI technologies.

This emerging technology AI can also help for scanning procedures and re-designing the work system of a contact with the patients, so the best quality and protection can be provided to them.

It can improve the working conditions by providing correct information of detection in CT and X-ray scans, which provides them with the finding of a disease and capacity to cure the disease.

10.13 CLASSIFICATION

According to the classification of these viruses, they are classified under their halo-like appearance, a main feature of replication. In the case of humans, it falls in one of the two types:

1. 1.229E-like.
2. OC43-like (Figure 10.12).

This paper represents the results which have affected people of older age to a large extent, rather than those of younger age, the main reason being their immune systems [5, 6].

According to health reports, the older people tend to have low immune systems, but the results could be seen that older people have beaten this coronavirus and are at safer and more stable condition than younger people [1].

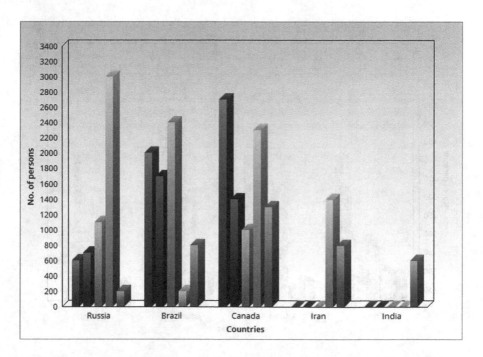

FIGURE 10.12   Position of Big Giants Countries conditions during coronavirus spread.

10.14   CURRENT REPORTS

As of now, dated 10 May 2020, 4,101,973 cases have been reported across the world, with 1,441,866 cases recovered [10]. According to current reports and statistics, 62,939 cases are reported in India, with 19,358 cases recovered [7] (Figure 10.13)

It concludes that neither are younger people safe from this virus, nor are older people the only ones to be affected. The people of the country need to be protected from its unusual behavior, and hence, must follow the rules provided by the World Health Organization (WHO) [7, 8].

German government update:

1. Confirmed cases – 67,366;deaths – 732.
2. 4 'High' coronavirus threat risk for Germany (Robert Koch Institute)
3. All states in Germany are affected –partial lockdown in German states; closure of non-essential shops, reduced public transport.
4. 4 Entry into EU of non-EU citizens has been banned for an initial period of 30 days with effect from 17 March 2020, with a few exceptions.
5. All passenger aircrafts to India are banned until 1830 hrs. GMT, 14 April2020 [5, 6] (Figure 10.14).

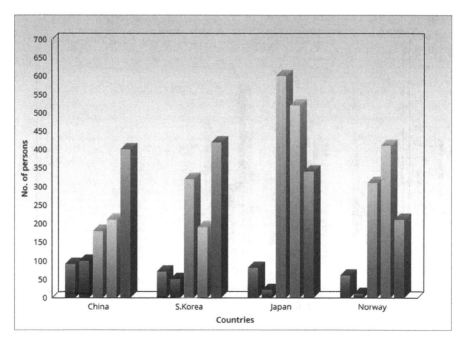

FIGURE 10.13   Position of countries after some time.

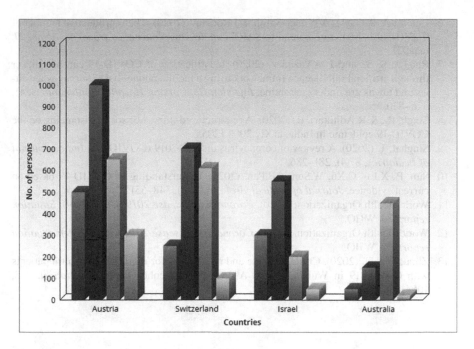

FIGURE 10.14   Position of countries where coronavirus cases increased after some time.

10.15   CONCLUSION

In this work, the major facts about the coronavirus and the consequences of the novel coronavirus, that has made the entire country suffer, have been discussed. The entire world is at stake due to red alert caused by increased number of cases of coronavirus in every country except the Antarctica. Due to these severe conditions, several measures have been taken into account to prevent countries from the severe effects of coronavirus. The details of the countries with statistical information are provided for clarity and better interpretation.

REFERENCES

1. Alimadadi, A., S.Aryal, I.Manandhar, P. B.Munroe, B.Joe, &X.Cheng. (2020). Artificial intelligence and machine learning to fight Covid-19. *Physiological Genomics*, 52(4), 200–202.
2. Bai, Y. et al. (2020). Presumed asymptomatic carrier transmission of COVID-19. *Jama*, 323(14), 1406–1407.
3. Dhama, K., et al. (2020). Coronavirus disease 2019–COVID-19. *Clinical Microbiology Reviews*, 33, e00028-20.
4. van der Hoek, L. et al. (2004). Identification of a new human coronavirus. *Nature medicine*, 10(4), 368–373.
5. Holmes, K. V. (2003). SARS-associated coronavirus. *New England Journal of Medicine*, 348(20), 1948–1951.

6. Liu, Y., A. A.Gayle, A.Wilder-Smith, &J.Rocklöv. (2020). The reproductive number of COVID-19 is higher compared to SARS coronavirus. *Journal of travel medicine*, 27, taaa021.

7. Rao, A. S. S., and J. A.Vazquez. (2020). Identification of COVID-19 can be quicker through artificial intelligence framework using a mobile phone–based survey when cities and towns are under quarantine. *Infection Control and Hospital Epidemiology*, 41, 826–830.

8. Singh, R., & R.Adhikari, R. (2020). Age-structured impact of social distancing on the COVID-19 epidemic in India. arXiv:2003.12055.

9. Singhal, T. (2020). A review of coronavirus disease-2019 (COVID-19). *Indian Journal of Pediatrics*, 87(4), 281–286.

10. Sun, P., X.Lu, C.Xu, W.Sun, &B.Pan. (2020). Understanding of COVID-19 based on current evidence. *Journal of medical virology*, 92(6), 548–551.

11. World Health Organization. (2020). *Coronavirus disease 2019 (COVID-19): Situation report*, 70. WHO.

12. World Health Organization. (2020). *Coronavirus disease 2019 (COVID-19): situation report*, 72. WHO.

13. Zhou, F. et al. (2020). Clinical course and risk factors for mortality of adult inpatients with COVID-19 in Wuhan, China: A retrospective cohort study. *The lancet*, 395, 1054–1062.

Index

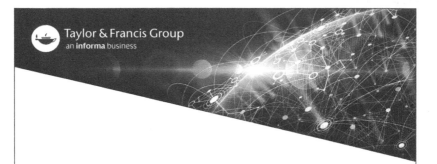